Common
Simple
Emergencies

Common
Simple
Emergencies

Philip M. Buttaravoli, MD, FACEP

Clinical Assistant Professor of Medicine (Emergency)
Georgetown University Medical Center
Chairman, Department of Emergency Medicine
Holy Cross Hospital, Silver Spring, Maryland

Thomas O. Stair, MD, FACEP

Assistant Professor of Medicine (Emergency)
Residency Director, Emergency Medicine
Georgetown University Medical Center
Washington, D.C.

Brady Communications Company, Inc.
A Prentice-Hall Publishing Company
Bowie, Maryland

Publishing Director: David Culverwell
Acquisitions Editor: Richard Weimer
Production Editor: Barbara Werner
Art Director: Don Sellers, AMI
Assistant Art Director: Bernard Vervin
Illustrator: Joseph Vitek
Text Designer: Michael Rogers

Typesetter: Phototype America, Cedar Falls, Iowa
Printer: R.R. Donnelley & Sons Co., Harrisonburg, Virginia

Library of Congress Cataloging in Publication Data

Buttaravoli, Philip M., 1945–
   Common simple emergencies.

   Includes index.
   1. Medical emergencies. I. Stair, Thomas O., 1950–   . II. Title.
[DNLM: 1. Emergencies. WB 105 B988c]
RC86.7.B88   1984   616'.025   84-12710
ISBN 0-89303-371-5

Prentice-Hall International, Inc., *London*
Prentice-Hall Canada, Inc., Scarborough, *Ontario*
Prentice-Hall of Australia, Pty., Ltd., *Sydney*
Prentice-Hall of India Private Limited, *New Delhi*
Prentice-Hall of Japan, Inc., *Tokyo*
Prentice-Hall of Southeast Asia Pte. Ltd., *Singapore*
Whitehall Books, Limited, Petone, *New Zealand*
Editora Prentice-Hall Do Brasil LTDA., *Rio de Janeiro*
Prentice-Hall Hispanoamericana, S.A., *Mexico*

Printed in the United States of America

85 86 87 88 89 90 91 92 93 94 95   1 2 3 4 5 6 7 8 9 10

To the best of our knowledge, recommended measures and dosages
herein are accurate and conform to prevalent standards at time of
publication. Please check the manufacturer's product information
sheet for any changes in the dosage schedule or contraindications.

The excellence of the practitioner depends far more upon good judgment than great learning.

Henry J. Bigelow, M.D.
Medical Education in America
(1871)

Dedication

To my wife, Susan, for her help and encouragement, and to my children, Pamela, Allison, and Frank, for the time I could not be with them

PMB

To my wife, Lucy Caldwell-Stair, and to my children, Peter and Rebecca, for their support and for the time I was away

TOS

Foreword

The management of common simple emergencies is a subject presently neglected in the curricula of most medical schools. Seldom does this material receive enough attention in the medical literature of today. The reason for this fact has always been unclear to me. When this question was raised during my undergraduate training, our professors were quick to assure us that this gap in our education would be filled during postgraduate years. The unfortunate truth is that graduate physicians are not adequately exposed to this valuable information, unless they receive their training from experienced emergency physicians.

Doctors Buttaravoli and Stair, by developing this practical, nicely illustrated, easy-to-read text, have served all practicing primary physicians well. It will prove to be extremely useful as a resource for undergraduate and graduate education in Emergency Medicine and should grace the library shelves of all hospital emergency departments, freestanding emergency centers, and similar ambulatory care settings.

John G. Wiegenstein, MD
Professor and Chief
Section of Emergency Medicine
Michigan State University

Preface

Patients seeking medical care for minor emergencies are often experiencing as much anguish and/or pain as those experiencing truly life- or limb-threatening emergencies. These patients trust that the physicians who treat them will be as caring, confident, and thorough in their duties as they would be when presented with a major medical problem.

On the other hand, it is quite possible to find today's young physicians either totally perplexed or falsely confident when confronted with a simple clinical problem that they just haven't seen before. The risk, then, is that they will lose rapport with the patient, be unable to provide any useful service to the patient, or, at worst, harm the patient.

It was with these problems in mind that in 1977 I began a lecture series for medical students at Georgetown University. *Common Simple Emergencies* grew out of that series.

Like the lectures, the book provides a review of the management of simple, acute, clinical problems and should assist the physician in dealing properly with these ubiquitous yet sometimes difficult situations.

I have found that, after providing patients with competent and sensitive care for the most minor and routine problems, I have been rewarded with gratitude no less intense than if I have performed major surgery.

Philip M. Buttaravoli, MD

This book is written for the health care professional just beginning work in an emergency department or clinic, to provide some guidance with the majority of patient problems which somehow are not covered in schools or textbooks. Even experienced practitioners, however, who have already learned many of these approaches from the oral traditions of medicine, or who have evolved their own methods, may benefit from comparing their approaches with those in this book.

The approaches to common simple emergencies described herein are sometimes unorthodox, but are the best we have come up with so far, and do reflect our own current clinical practices. Whenever possible, our recommendations are based on our own or others' clinical research. Where formal studies were unavailable, as was often the case, we fell back on our clinical experience. We have avoided, as far as possible, promulgating unexamined medical traditions or repeating "the way we've always done it."

Much more basic and clinical research remains to be done on the management of common simple emergencies, and we welcome contributions from our readers concerning topics, approaches, insights, clinical trials, quantification, and analysis.

Thomas O. Stair, MD

Acknowledgments

Thanks

to Drs Claude Cadoux, David B. Doman, Roy Farrell, Douglas Greer, Pierre d'Hemecourt, Lester Marion, William Maxfield, Hubert Mickel, J. Douglas White, and John Wiegenstein for reviewing portions of the manuscript;

to Tamra Walton, Joe Sirvan, Joan Swift, and Chris Spears for help with typing of the manuscript;

to Allison and Frank Buttaravoli and Rebecca and Peter Stair for hours of patient posing;

to Joe Vitek, for his expert illustrations;

to our editor, Barbara Werner, for her patience and good humor.

And special thanks to Judy and Amen Hillow.

Contents

1 NEUROLOGIC

Vasovagal syncope (faint, swoon)   1
Hyperventilation   2
Minor head trauma ("concussion")   5
Seizures (convulsions, fits)   7
Hysterical coma or seizure   9
Dystonic drug reaction   12
Tension headache   14
Migraine headache   17
Polymyalgia rheumatica   19
Weakness   20
Vertigo ("dizzy, lightheaded")   22
Bell's palsy (facial weakness)   27

2 OPHTHALMOLOGIC

Periobital ecchymosis (black eye)   29
Conjunctivitis   31
Iritis   32
Conjunctival foreign body   35
Corneal foreign body   38
Corneal abrasion   40
Periorbital and conjunctival edema   42
Subconjunctival hemorrhage   44
Ultraviolet keratoconjunctivitis   45
Hordeolum (sty)   46
Contact lens overwear   47
Removal of dislocated contact lens   49
Removal of contact lens in unconscious patient   50

3 EAR/NOSE/THROAT

Cerumen impaction (ear wax blockage)   53
Otitis externa (swimmer's ear)   55
Perforated tympanic membrane   58
Foreign body—ear   59
Serous otitis media   62
Split earlobe   65
Epistaxis (nosebleed)   66
Nasal foreign bodies   69
Nasal fractures   72
Sinusitis   73
Pharyngitis (sore throat)   75
Foreign body in throat   78
Mononucleosis (glandular fever)   80

4   ORAL/DENTAL

Temporomandibular joint arthritis   83
Jaw dislocation   86
Lacerations of the mouth   87
Aphthous ulcer (canker sore)   90
Oral herpes simplex (cold sore)   90
Sialolithiasis (salivary duct stones)   91
Dental trauma   94
Bleeding after dental surgery   95
Dental pain post extraction (dry socket)   96
Dental pain—pulpitis   97
Dental pain—abscess   98
Dental pain—pericoronitis   99
Gingivitis   100
Oral candidiasis (thrush)   101

5   PULMONARY/THORACIC

Upper respiratory infection (cold)   103
Rib fracture/costochondral separation   105
Costochrondritis   108
Xyphoiditis   109
Tear gas exposure   110
Inhalation injury   111

6   GASTROINTESTINAL

Singultus (hiccups)   115
Esophageal food bolus obstruction (steakhouse syndrome)   116
Swallowed foreign body   119
Innocuous ingestions   120
Food poisoning—staphylococcal   121
Diarrhea   123
Gas pain and constipation   125
Enterobiasis (threadworms, pinworms)   126
Hemorrhoids (piles)   127
Rectal foreign body   129

7   UROLOGIC

Lower urinary tract infection (cystitis)   135
Upper urinary tract infection (pyelonephritis)   137
Colorful urine   138
Urethritis (drip)   139
Gonorrhea (clap)   140
Genital herpes simplex   142
Epididymitis   143
Prostatitis   145

Urinary retention   146
Phimosis and paraphimosis   148

8   GYNECOLOGIC

Dysmenorrhea (menstrual cramps)   151
Vaginal bleeding   152
Vaginitis   154
Vaginal foreign bodies   156
Bartholin abscess   157

9   MUSCULOSKELETAL

Cervical strain (whiplash)   161
Torticollis (wry neck)   162
Acute lumbar strain (low back pain, facet syndrome)   165
Coccyx fracture (tailbone fracture)   166
Fibromyalgia (trigger points)   168
Acute monarticular arthritis   170
Podagra (acute gouty arthritis)   173
Bursitis   174
Ligament sprains and joint capsule injuries   176
Muscle strains and tears   177
Traumatic effusion   178
Subluxation of the head of the radius (nursemaid's elbow)   180
Radial head fracture   182
Radial neuropathy   184
Cheiralgia paresthetica (handcuff neuropathy)   186
Carpal tunnel syndrome   188
Ganglion cysts   190
Scaphoid (carpal navicular) fracture   191
Skipole or gamekeeper's thumb   193
Finger (PIP joint) dislocation   194
Extensor tendon avulsion—distal phalanx (baseball or mallet finger)   196
Plantaris tendon rupture   198
Broken toe   200

10   SOFT TISSUE

Superficial fingertip avulsion   203
Nail root dislocation   205
Finger or toenail avulsion   207
Ring removal   209
Nailbed laceration   212
Subungual hematoma   214
Subungual ecchymosis   216
Foreign body beneath nail   217
Paronychia   219

Bicycle spoke injury   222
Needle (foreign body) in foot   223
Puncture wounds   227
Minor impalement injuries   229
Fishhook removal   231
Traumatic tattoos and abrasions   233
Bites   235

11   SKIN

Rhus dermatitis (poison ivy)   239
Sunburn   240
Partial thickness (2nd degree) burns and tar burns   241
Frostbite and frostnip   244
Hymenoptera envenomations (bee stings)   246
Superficial sliver   247
Pencil point puncture   249
Metallic foreign body   251
Tick removal   253
Cutaneous abscess or pustule   256
Erystipelas, cellulitis, and lymphangitis   258
Pyogenic granuloma   259
Zipper caught on penis or chin   260
Contusions (bruises)   262
Urticaria (hives)   264
Pityriasis rosea   265
Tinea (athlete's foot, ringworm)   267
Herpes zoster (shingles)   269
Pediculosis (lice, crabs)   271
Scabies   273
Impetigo   274
Diaper rash   275

12   PROPHYLAXIS

Tetanus prophylaxis   277
Rabies prophylaxis   278
Hepatitis A prophylaxis   280
Hepatitis B prophylaxis   280
Needlestick   281

APPENDIX

Digital nerve block   283
A simple finger tip dressing   284
Complete eye exam   285
Certified regional poison centers   287

INDEX   293

Neurologic

Vasovagal Syncope (Faint, swoon)

Presentation:

First, there is a period of sympathetic tone, with increased pulse and blood pressure, in anticipation of some stressful incident, such as bad news, an upsetting sight, or a painful procedure. Immediately following the stressful occurrence, there is a precipitous drop in sympathetic tone, pulse and blood pressure, causing the victim to fall down and/or lose consciousness.

Transient bradycardia and few clonic limb jerks may accompany vasovagal syncope, but there are usually no sustained arrhythmias or seizures, incontinence, tongue biting, or injuries beyond a contusion or laceration from the fall.

Ordinarily, the victim spontaneously revives after spending a few minutes supine, and suffers no sequelae.

The whole process may transpire in the ED, or a patient may have fainted elsewhere, in which case the diagnostic challenge is to reconstruct what happened and rule out other causes of syncope.

What to do:

- Arrange for patients, family, and friends anticipating unpleasant experiences in the ED to sit or lie down and be constantly attended.
- If someone faints in the ED, catch him so he is not injured in the fall, lie him supine on the floor for 5–10 minutes, protect his airway, record several sets of vital signs, and be ready to proceed with resuscitation if the episode turns out to be more than a simple vasovagal syncope.
- If a patient is brought to the ED following a faint elsewhere, ask about the setting, precipitating factors, descriptions of several eyewitnesses, and sequence of recovery. Be alert for evidence of seizures (p 7), hysteria (p 9), and hyperventilation (p 2). Record

several sets of vital signs, including orthostatic changes, and examine carefully for signs of trauma and neurological residua.

- After full recovery, explain to the patient that this is a common physiological reaction and how, in future recurrences, he can recognize the early lightheadedness, and prevent a full swoon by lying down or putting his head between his knees.

What not to do:

- Do not let families stand for bad news, allow parents to stand while watching their children being sutured, or let patients stand for shots or venipuncture.
- Do not traumatize the faint victim with ammonia capsules, cold water dousing, or slapping.
- Do not allow patients to feel embarrassed or belittled because they fainted.

Discussion:

Vasovagal syncope is a common occurrence in the ED. Observation of the entire sequence makes the diagnosis, but, better yet, the whole reaction can usually be easily prevented.

It should be noted that although most patients suffer no sequelae, vasovagal syncope with prolonged asystole can produce seizures as well as rare incidents of death. In addition, it should be remembered that the differential diagnosis of a loss of consciousness is extensive and therefore loss of consciousness in the emergency department should not immediately be assumed to be due to vasovagal syncope.

Hyperventilation

Presentation:

The patient is anxious and complains of shortness of breath and an inability to fill the lungs adequately. A patient may also have palpitations, chest or abdominal pain, and tingling or numbness around the mouth and fingers, or possibly even flexor spasm of the hands and feet. His respiratory volume is increased, which may be apparent by an increased respiratory rate, or only be an increased tidal volume or frequent sighing. The remainder of the physical examination is normal. The patient's history may reveal an obvious precipitating emotional cause (such as having been caught stealing or being in the midst of a family quarrel).

What to do:

- Perform a brief physical examination, checking especially that the patient's mental status is good, there is no unusual breath odor, there are good, equal excursion and breath sounds in both sides of the chest, and there is no swelling or inflammation of the legs.
- Explain to the patient the cycle in which rapid, deep breathing can cause physical symptoms upsetting enough to cause further rapid, deep breathing. Repeat a cadence ("in . . . out . . . in . . .") to help him voluntarily slow his breathing, or have him voluntarily hold his breath for a while.
- If he cannot reduce his ventilatory rate and volume, provide a paper bag or length of tubing through which to breathe. This will allow him to continue moving a large quantity of air, but provide air rich in carbon dioxide, allowing the blood Pco_2 to rise towards normal. Carbogen (5% CO_2) may also be used, if available. Administration of 50 – 100mg of hydroxyzine (Vistaril) im often helps to calm the patient.
- If you cannot reverse these symptoms and reduce respiratory effect in this manner in 15–20 minutes, you should double-check the diagnosis by obtaining arterial blood gases, looking for a metabolic acidosis or hypoxia indicative of underlying disease.
- Reexamine the patient after hyperventilation is controlled.
- Make sure the patient understands the hyperventilation syndrome and knows some strategies for breaking the cycle next time. (It may be valuable to have him reproduce the symptoms voluntarily.) Arrange for followup as needed.

What not to do:

Do not miss the true medical emergencies which also present as hyperventilation, including: pneumothorax, pneumonia, pulmonary embolus, diabetic ketoacidosis, salicylate overdose, sepsis, uremia, and CVA.

Discussion:

The acute metabolic alkalosis of hyperventilation causes transient imbalances of calcium, potassium, and perhaps other ions, with the net effect of increasing the irritability and spontaneous depolarization of excitable muscles and nerves.

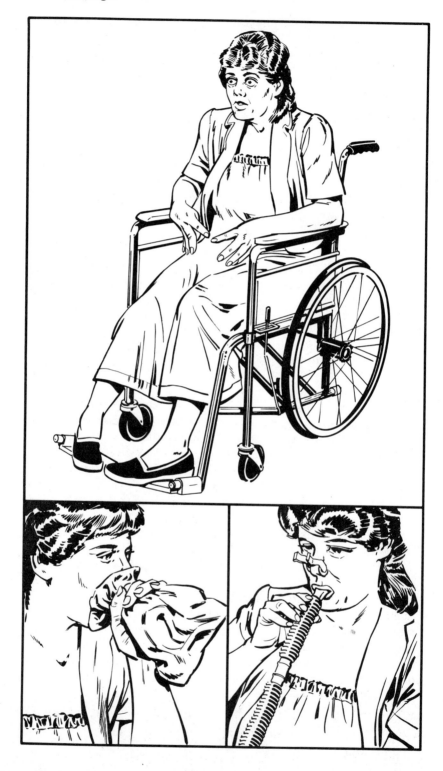

First-time victims of the hyperventilation syndrome are the most apt to visit the ED, and this is an excellent time to educate them about its pathophysiology and the prevention of recurrence. Repeat visitors may be overly excitable or may have emotional problems and need counseling.

Minor Head Trauma ("Concussion")

Presentation:

A patient is brought to the ED after suffering a blow to the head. There may or may not be a laceration, scalp hematoma, headache, transient sleepiness and/or nausea, but there was NO loss of consciousness, amnesia for the injury or preceding events, seizure, neurological changes, or disorientation. The patient or family may express concern about a "mild concussion," the possibility of a skull fracture, or a rapidly developing scalp hematoma or "goose egg."

What to do:

- Corroborate and record the history from witnesses. Ascertain why the patient was injured (was there a seizure or sudden weakness?) and rule out particularly dangerous types of head trauma. (A blow by a brick or hammer is more likely to produce a depressed skull fracture.)
- Perform and record a physical examination of the head, looking for signs of a skull fracture, such as hemotympanum or bony depression, and examine the neck for spasm, bony tenderness, rage of motion, and other signs of associated injury.
- Perform and record a neurological examination, with special attention to mental status, cranial nerves, strength, and deep tendon reflexes to all four limbs.
- If the history or physical examination suggests there could be a clinically significant skull fracture, obtain skull x rays. Criteria for obtaining skull x rays include: documented loss of consciousness, amnesia, a blow by a heavy object, suspected skull penetration, palpable depression, CSF leaking from nose or ear, blood behind the TM or over the mastoid (Battle's sign), bilateral periorbital ecchymoses (raccoon eyes), stupor, coma, or any focal neurological sign.
- If there is no clinical indication for skull films, explain to the patient and concerned family and friends why x rays are not

being ordered. Many patients expect x rays, but will gladly forego them once you explain they are of little value.

- Explain to the patient and responsible family or friends that the more important possible sequelae of head trauma are not diagnoses with x rays, but by noting certain signs and symptoms as they occur later. Make sure that they understand (and write down) that any abnormal behavior, increasing drowsiness or difficulty in rousing the patient, headache, neck stiffness, vomiting, visual problems, weakness, or seizures are signals to return to the ED immediately.

What not to do:

- Do not skimp on the neurological examination or its documentation.
- Do not be reassured by negative skull films, which do not rule out intracranial bleeding or edema.

Discussion:

The risks of late neurological sequelae (subdural hematoma, seizure disorder, meningitis, post-concussion syndrome, etc.) make good followup essential after any head trauma; but the vast majority of patients without findings on initial examination do well.

It is probably unwise to describe to the patient all of the subtle possible long-term effects of head trauma, because many may be induced by suggestion. Concentrate on making sure all understand the danger signs to watch for over the next few days.

The old practice of routinely x raying all head trauma is slowly dying out. Indeed, any patient satisfying the criteria outlined above for skull x rays might be better examined by computed tomography, if available, because CT shows intracranial bleeding and edema invisible on plain films.

A large scalp hematoma may have a soft central area which mimics a depression in the skull when palpated directly, but allows palpation of the underlying skull when pushed to one side. Cold packs may be recommended to reduce the swelling, and the patient may be reassured that the hematoma will resolve over days to weeks.

Seizures (Convulsions, fits)

Presentation:

The patient may be found in the street, the hospital, or the emergency room. The patient may be complaining of an "aura," feel he is "about to have a seizure," experience a brief petit mal "absence," the repetitive stereotypical behavior of continuous partial seizures, the whole-body tonic stiffness or clonic jerking of grand mal seizures, or simply be found in the gradual recovery of the postictal phase. The only true emergency is the patient experiencing a grand mal seizure.

What to do:

- If the patient is having a grand mal seizure, stand by him for a few minutes until his thrashing subsides, to guard against injury or airway obstruction. Usually only suctioning or turning the patient on his side is required, but breathing will be uncoordinated until the tonic-clonic phase is over.

  Watch the pattern of the seizure for clues to the etiology. (Did clonus start in one place and "march" out to the rest of the body? Did the eyes deviate one way throughout the seizure? Did the whole body participate?)

  If the seizure lasts more than two minutes, or recurs before the patient regains consciousness, it has overwhelmed the brain's natural buffers and may require drugs to stop. This is defined as status epilepticus, and is best treated with diazepam (Valium) 5–10mg iv, followed by gradual loading with iv phenytoin.

- If the patient arrives postictal, examine him thoroughly for injuries and record a complete neurological examination (the results of which are apt to be bizarre). Repeat the neurological exam periodically. If the patient is indeed recovering, you may be able to obviate much of the diagnostic workup by waiting until he is lucid enough to give a history.

- If the patient arrives awake and oriented following an alleged seizure, corroborate the history through witnesses or the presence of injuries like a scalp laceration or a bitten tongue. Doubt a grand mal seizure without a prolonged postictal recovery period.

- If the patient has a previous history of seizure disorder, or is taking anticonvulsant medications, check old records, speak to his physician, find out whether he has been worked up for an etiology, look for reasons for this relapse (e.g., infection, ethanol, lack of sleep), and draw blood for levels of anticonvulsants.

- If the seizure is clearly related to alcohol withdrawal, ascertain why the patient reduced his consumption. He might be broke, be suffering from pancreatitis or gastritis that requires further evaluation and treatment, or have decided to dry out completely. If the last, his withdrawal should be medically supervised, and covered with benzodiazepines (e.g., Librium or Valium).

    Be careful not to assume an alcoholic etiology. Ethanol abusers sustain more head trauma and seizure disorders than the population at large. Many emergency physicians presumptively treat alcohol withdrawal symptoms with 25gm glucose, 100mg thiamine, and 2gm magnesium iv.

- If the seizure is a new event, make arrangements for a workup, including an EEG. This need not require hospitalization, but if discharged, the patient should be loaded with 18mg/kg of phenytoin (over ½ hour iv, or over 6 hours po) to protect him from further seizures. If possible, check Dilantin level before giving this loading dose.

What not to do:

- Do not stick anything in the mouth of a seizing patient. The ubiquitous padded throat sticks may be nice for a patient to hold and bite on at the first sign of a seizure, but do nothing to protect his airway, and are ineffective when the jaw is clenched.
- Do not rush to give intravenous diazepam to a seizing patient. Most seizures stop in a few minutes. It is diagnostically useful to see how the seizure resolves on its own; also, the patient will awaken sooner if he has not been medicated. Reserve diazepam for genuine status epilepticus.
- Do not treat alcohol withdrawal seizures with phenobarbital or phenytoin. Both lack efficacy (and necessity, since the problem is self-limiting) and can themselves produce withdrawal seizures.
- Do not rule out alcohol withdrawal seizures on the basis of a toxic serum ethanol level. The patient may actually be withdrawing from a yet higher baseline.
- Do not be fooled by pseudoseizures. Even patients with genuine epilepsy occasionally fake seizures for various reasons, and an exceptional performer can be convincing. Amateurs may be roused with ammonia or smelling salts, but few can simulate the fluctuating neurological abnormalities of the postictal state, and probably no one can produce the pronounced metabolic acidosis of a grand mal seizure.
- Do not let a seizure victim drive home.

Discussion:

Grand mal seizures are frightening, and inspire observers to "do something," but usually all that is necessary is to stand by and prevent the patient from injuring himself.

The age of the patient makes some difference as to the probable underlying etiology of a first seizure and therefore makes some difference in disposition. In the 12–20-year-old patient, the seizure is probably "idiopathic," although other causes are certainly possible. In the 40-year-old patient with a first seizure, one needs to exclude neoplasm, post-traumatic epilepsy, or withdrawal. In the 65-year-old patient with a first seizure, cerebrovascular insufficiency must also be considered. Such a patient should be treated and worked up with the possibility of an impending stroke, in addition to the other possible causes.

For these reasons, a patient with a first seizure, who is 30 years old or older, needs to have a CT scan, preferably while in the ED. A non-contrast study can be obtained initially. If there are abnormalities present or if there are still suspicions of a focal abnormality, a contrast study can be obtained at the same time or later, whichever is convenient.

Also, patients should be discharged for outpatient care, only if there is full recovery of neurological function, with a full loading dose of phenytoin, and with clear arrangements for follow-up and/or return to the ED if another seizure occurs.

The traditional laboratory workup for an etiology (urinalysis, blood counts, glucose, BUN, blood gases, and ECG) is reasonably effective and efficient. Skull films should be reserved for clinically evident head trauma, and an EEG can usually be done electively, except in status epilepticus. A toxic screen may be needed to detect the many overdoses that can present as seizures, such as amoxapine, amphetamines, cocaine, lidocaine, and phencyclidine.

Hysterical Coma or Seizure

Presentation:

The patient is unresponsive and brought to the emergency department on a stretcher. There is usually a history of recent emotional upset an unexpected death in the family, breakup of a close relationship. The patient may be lying still on the stretcher or demonstrating bizarre posturing or even seizure-like activity. The patient's general color and vital signs are normal, without any evidence of airway obstruction. Commonly, the patient will be fluttering his eyelids or will resist having his eyes opened. A striking finding is that the patient may hold his breath when the examiner breaks an ammonia capsule over the patient's mouth and nose (real coma victims usually move the head or do nothing). A classic finding is that when the patient's apparently flaccid arm is released over his face, it does not fall on the face, but drops off to the side. The patient may show remarkably little response to painful stimuli, but there should be no true focal neurologic findings and the remainder of the physical exam should be normal.

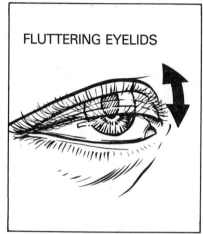

FLUTTERING EYELIDS

What to do:

- Do a complete physical exam. Patients sometimes react with hysterical coma under stress of illness or injury.
- When there is significant emotional stress involved, administer a mild tranquilizing agent such as hydroxyzine pamoate (Vistaril) 50–100mg im.
- Do not allow any visitors and place the patient in a quiet observation area, minimizing any stimulation until he "awakens." Check vital signs every 30 minutes.
- When the patient becomes more responsive, re-examine him, obtain a more complete history, and offer him followup care, including psychological support if appropriate.
- If the patient is not awake, alert, and oriented after about 90 minutes, begin a more comprehensive medical workup.

What not to do:

- Do not get angry with the patient and torture him with painful stimuli in an attempt to make him "wake up."
- Do not perform an expensive workup routinely.
- Do not ignore or release the patient who has not fully recovered. Instead, he must be admitted to the hospital and evaluated for an underlying medical problem.

Discussion:

True hysterical coma is substantially an unconscious act that the patient cannot control. Antagonizing the patient often prolongs the

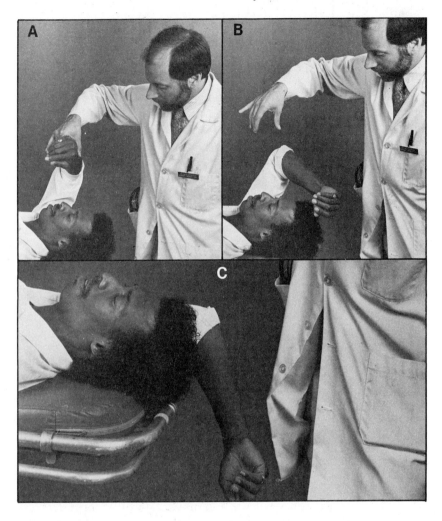

condition, while ignoring him seems to take the spotlight off his peculiar behavior, allowing him to recover.

Some psychomotor seizures are difficult to diagnose and might be labeled hysterical. If the diagnosis is not obviously hysteria, the patient might need an EEG during sleep and deserves a referral to a neurologist.

Dystonic Drug Reaction

Presentation:

Often there is no history offered at all—the patient may not be able to speak, may not be aware he took any phenothiazines or butyrophenones (e.g., Haldol has been used to cut heroin), may not admit he takes psychotropic medication, or may not make the connection between symptoms and drug (e.g., one dose of Compazine given for vomiting).

Acute dystonias usually present with one or more of the following symptoms:

- buccolingual—protruding, or pulling sensation of tongue
- torticollic—twisted neck, or facial muscle spasm
- oculogyric—roving or deviated gaze
- tortipelvic—abdominal rigidity and pain
- opisthotonic—spasm of the entire body

These acute dystonias can resemble partial seizures, the posturing of psychosis, or the spasms of tetanus, strychnine poisoning, or electrolyte imbalances. More chronic neurologic side effects of phenothiazines, including the restlessness of akathisia, tardive dyskinesias, and Parkinsonism, do not usually respond as dramatically to drug treatment as the acute dystonias.

What to do:

- Give 2mg of benztropine (Cogentin) or 50mg of diphenhydramine (Benadryl) iv, and watch for improvement of the dystonia over the next five minutes. This step is both therapeutic and diagnostic. Benztropine produces fewer side effects (mostly drowsiness), and may be slightly more effective, but diphenhydramine is more likely to be on hand in the ED.
- Instruct the patient to discontinue the offending drug, and arrange for followup if medications must be adjusted. If the culprit is long-acting, prescribe benztropine (Cogentin) 2mg or diphenhydramine (Benadryl) 25mg po q6h for 24 hours to prevent a relapse.

What not to do:

- Do not persist with treatment in the face of a questionable response or no response, but get on with the workup to find another etiology for the dystonia (tetanus, seizures, hypomagnesemia, hypocalcemia, alkalosis, muscle disease, etc.).
- Do not use intravenous diazepam first, because it relaxes spasms due to other etiologies, and thus leaves the diagnosis unclear.

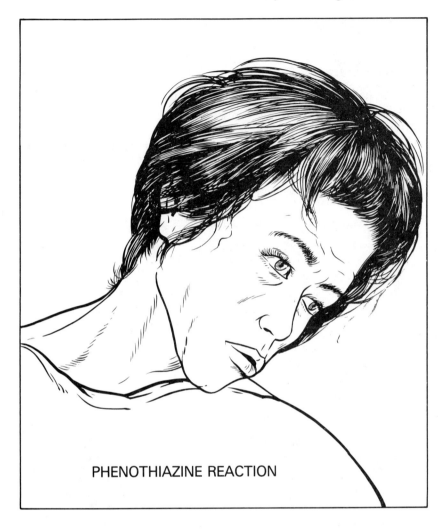

PHENOTHIAZINE REACTION

Discussion:

The extrapyramidal motor system depends on excitatory cholinergic neurotransmitters and inhibitory dopaminergic neurotransmittors, the latter susceptible to blockage by phenothiazine and butyrophenone medications. Anticholinergic medications restore the excitatory-inhibitory balance.

One intravenous dose of benztropine or diphenhydramine is relatively innocuous and rapidly diagnostic, and is probably justified as an initial step in any patient with a dystonic reaction.

Tension Headache

Presentation:

The patient complains of a dull, steady pain, described as an ache, pressure, throb, or constricting band, located anywhere from eyes to occiput, perhaps including the neck or shoulders. Most commonly, the headache develops near the end of the day, or after some particular stress. The pain may improve with rest, aspirin, acetaminophen, or other medications. The physical exam will be unremarkable except for cranial or posterior cervical muscle tenderness.

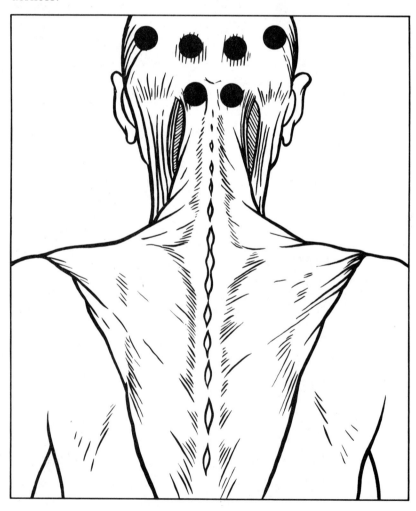

What to do:

- Perform a complete general history (including environmental factors and foods which precede the headaches) and physical examination (including a neurological examination).
- If the patient complains of sudden onset of the "worst headache of my life," accompanied by any change in mental status, weakness, vomiting, seizures, stiff neck, or persistent neurologic abnormalities, suspect a cerebrovascular cause, especially a subarachnoid hemorrhage, intracranial hemorrhage, or arteriovenous malformation. The best diagnostic test for these is computed tomography, but when CT is not available and the patient does not have papilledema or other signs of increased intracranial pressure, rule out these problems with a lumbar puncture.
- If the headache is accompanied by fever and stiff neck, or change in mental status, you need to rule out bacterial meningitis as soon as possible.
- If the headache was preceded by ophthalmic or neurologic symptoms, now resolving, suggestive of a migraine headache, you may want to try ergotamine therapy (see p 17). If vasospastic symptoms persist into the headache phase, the etiology may still be a migraine, but it becomes more important to rule out other cerebrovascular causes.
- If the headache follows prolonged reading, driving, or television watching, and decreased visual acuity is improved by viewing through a pinhole, the headache may be due to a defect in optical refraction, curable with new lenses.
- If the temples are tender, check for visual defects and myalgias that accompany temporal arteritis (see p 19).
- If there is a history of recent dental work or grinding of teeth, tenderness anterior to the tragus, or crepitus on motion of the jaw, suspect arthritis of the temperomandibular joint (see p 83).
- If there is fever, tenderness to percussion over the frontal or maxillary sinuses, or purulent drainage visible in the nose, consider an upright Water's view to demonstrate sinusitis (see p 73).
- If pain radiates to the ear, be sure to inspect and palpate the teeth, which are a common site of referred pain.
- Finally, after checking for all these other causes of headache, palpate the temporalis, occipitalis, and other muscles of the calvarium and neck, looking for areas of tenderness and spasm which usually accompany muscle tension headaches. Keep an eye out for especially tender "trigger points" which may resolve with gentle pressure or massage.

- Prescribe anti-inflammatory analgesics (e.g., aspirin, ibuprofen), recommend rest, and have the patient try cool compresses and massage of any trigger points.
- Explain the etiology and treatment of muscle spasm of the head and neck.
- Volunteer the information that you see no evidence of other serious disease (if this is true); especially that a brain tumor is unlikely. (Often this is a fear which is never voiced.)
- Arrange for followup. Instruct the patient to return to the ED or contact his own physician if symptoms change or worsen.

What not to do:

- Do not berate the patient for coming to the ED with "nothing but a tension headache."
- Do not discharge without followup instructions. Many serious illnesses begin with a minor cephalgia, and patients may postpone urgent care in the belief that they have been definitively diagnosed on the first visit.
- Do not miss subarachnoid hemorrhage and meningitis. (If you are not obtaining a majority of negative CTs and LPs, you may not be looking hard enough.)

Discussion:

Headaches are common and most are benign, but any headache brought to medical attention deserves a thorough evaluation. Screening tests are of little value—a laborious history and physical examination are required. Common causes of headache include viral myalgias, caffeine withdrawal, food intolerance, hypertension and carbon monoxide exposure. Uncommon but important causes include glaucoma and tic douloureux.

Tension headache is not a wastebasket diagnosis of exclusion but a specific diagnosis, confirmed by palpating tenderness in craniocervical muscles. The first priority, however, is to rule out life-threatening causes of headache such as CVA or meningitis. Focal tenderness over the greater occipital nerves (C2, 3) can be associated with an occipital neuralgia or occipital headache, and be secondary to cervical radiculopathy from cervical spondylosis. These tend to occur in older patients and should not be confused with tension headache.

Tension headache is often dignified with the diagnosis of "migraine" without any evidence of a vascular etiology, and is often treated with minor tranquilizers, which may or may not help. Remember to probe for the patient's hidden agenda. "Headache" may often be the justification for seeing a physician when some other physical, emotional, or social concern is actually the patient's major problem.

Migraine Headache

Presentation:

The patient comes to the ED with a steady, severe, pain in the left or right side of the head, following ophthalmic or neurologic symptoms which resolved as the headache developed. Scintillating, castellated scotomata in the visual field corresponding to the side of the subsequent headache are the classic aura, but transient weakness, vertigo, or ataxia are more likely to bring patients to the ED. Unlike other headaches, migraines are especially likely to awaken one in the morning. There may be a family or personal history of similar headaches as well.

What to do:

- If the pain is severe, begin with narcotic analgesics (e.g., meperidine, 50–100mg im, perhaps coupled with hydroxyzine or promethazine 25–50mg im to reduce nausea and prolong analgesia) and let the patient lie down in a dark, quiet room. It can be rather cruel to attempt a complete history and physical examination (and unrealistic to expect the patient to cooperate) before achieving some relief of pain.
- If the patient has not already tried any vasoconstrictive medications, such as ergotamine and caffeine, they can still be used. Although most effective when taken early, during the vasospastic aura and before the vasodilatory headache, they often provide some relief even after the headache is underway. If the patient can take medication orally, try tablets of ergotamine 2mg and caffeine 100mg (Cafergot), two at the first sign of the aura, then one every half hour up to a total day's dose of 6 tablets. If nausea and vomiting prevent oral medication, Cafergot is also available in rectal suppositories at the same dosage, but one or two suppositories are usually sufficient to relieve a headache. Ergotamine can also be given intramuscularly, in a dose of 0.5mg.
- After 15–20 minutes, when the patient is feeling a little better, undertake the history and physical examination. If there are persistent changes in mental status or neurological examination, a stiff neck, or fever, proceed with computed tomography and/or lumbar puncture to rule out intracranial hemorrhage or infection as the actual cause of the "migraine."
- If the presentation is indeed consistent with a migraine, allow the patient to sleep in the ED, undisturbed except for a brief neurological examination each hour. Typically, the patient will awaken after a few hours, with the headache much improved, and no neurological residua.

- Discharge the patient with a prescription for ergotamine and instructions for aborting the next attack. Provide direction to return to the ED for any change or worsening of the usual migraine pattern, and arrangements for medical followup. First-time migraine attacks deserve a thorough elective neurological evaluation to establish the diagnosis.

What not to do:

- Do not prescribe medications containing egotamine, caffeine, or barbiturates for continual prophylaxis. They will not be effective this way, and withdrawal from these drugs may produce headaches.
- Do not omit followup, especially for first attacks.
- Do not miss meningitis or a CVA, which may deteriorate rapidly undiagnosed. (If the aura is invariable and the pain always on the same side, the "migraine" may in reality be an arteriovenous malformation or other structural defect.)

Discussion:

Even more characteristic of migraine than the aura is the unilateral pain ("migraine" is a corruption of "hemicranium"). The pathophysiology is probably unilateral cerebral vasospasm (producing the neurological symptoms of the aura) followed by vasodilation (producing the headache). Neurologic symptoms may persist into the headache phase, but the longer they persist, the less likely they are due to the migraine. Cluster headaches, probably also of vascular origin, are characterized by lacrimation, rhinorrhea, and clustering in time, but the treatment of an attack is usually the same as for migraines.

One should be very cautious in the use of ergot preparations in any patient who has focal weakness or sensory deficits as part of the prodrome of their headache. It is possible to precipitate an ischemic infarct in such patients by using ergot preparations, which act by causing vasoconstriction.

Patients with aneurysms or A-V malformations can present clinically as migraine patients. If there is something different about the severity or nature of *this* headache, one must think of the possibility of a subarachnoid hemorrhage. Also, headaches, that are always on the same side and in the same location are very suspicious for an underlying structural lesion (e.g., aneurysm, AV malformation).

Many patients seeking narcotics have learned that faking a migraine headache is even easier than faking a ureteral stone, but they usually do not follow through the typical course of falling asleep after a shot of Demerol and waking up a few hours later with pain relieved. It is a good policy to limit narcotics to one or two shots for migraine headaches, and not prescribe oral narcotics from the ED.

Another good treatment for a severe migraine headache is giving 50–75mg (1mg/kg) of chlorpromazine (Thorazine) im, which is usually sufficiently sedative to allow the patient to go to sleep. Most migraine headaches will be much relieved after an hour or two of sleep.

Polymyalgia Rheumatica

Presentation:

An elderly patient (more commonly female) complains of a week or two of morning stiffness, which may interfere with her ability to rise from bed, but improves during the day. She may ascribe her problem to muscle weakness or joint pains, but physical examination discloses that symmetrical pain and tenderness of neck, shoulder, and hip muscles are the actual source of any "weakness." There may be some mild arthritis of several peripheral joints, but the rest of the physical examination is negative.

What to do:

- Perform a complete history and physical examination, particularly of the cervical and lumbar spines and nerve roots (strength, sensation, and deep tendon reflexes in the distal limbs should be intact with PMR). Confirm the diagnosis of PMR by palpating tender shoulder muscles (perhaps also hips, and, less commonly, neck).
- Confirm the diagnosis by obtaining an erythrocyte sedimentation rate, which should be in the 30–100mm/hour range. (An especially high ESR, over 100/hour suggests more severe autoimmune disease or malignancy.)
- Mild and borderline cases may respond with non-steroidal anti-inflammatory medications (e.g., Motrin). More severe cases will respond to prednisone 20–60mg qd within a week or two, after which the dose should be tapered. Failure to respond to corticosteroid therapy suggests some other diagnosis.
- Explain the syndrome to the patient and arrange for followup.

What not to do:

- Do not miss temporal arteritis, a common component of the polymyalgia rheumatica syndrome, and a clue to the existence of ophthalmic and cerebral arteritis, which can have dire neurological consequences. Palpate the temporal arteries for tenderness, swelling, or induration, and ask about transient neurological signs.
- Do not postpone diagnosis or treatment of temporal arteritis pending results of a temporal artery biopsy. The arteritis typically skips areas, making biopsy an insensitive diagnostic procedure.

Discussion:

Stiffness, pain, and weakness are common complaints in older patients, but polymyalgia rheumatica may respond dramatically to treatment. Rheumatoid arthritis produces morning stiffness, but is usually present in more peripheral joints, and without muscle tenderness. Polymyositis is usually characterized by increased serum muscle enzymes with a normal ESR, and may include a skin rash (dermatomyositis). Often, a therapeutic trial of prednisone helps make the diagnosis.

Weakness

Presentation:

An older patient comes to the emergency department or is brought by family, complaining of "weakness," or an inability to carry on his usual activities or care for himself.

What to do:

- Work at obtaining as much history as possible. Speak to available family members or friends, as well as the patient, and ask for details: Is the patient weak before certain activities? (suggestive of depression); is the weakness located in the limb girdles (suggestive of polymyalgia rheumatica, or myopathy); is the weakness mostly in the distal muscles? (neuropathy); is the weakness brought out by repetitive actions? (myasthenia gravis).

- Obtain a thorough medical history and physical examination, including a review of systems (headaches, weight loss, cold intolerance, appetite, bowel habits), strength of all muscle groups (graded on a scale of 1–5), deep tendon reflexes, and neurological status.
- Obtain a spectrum of laboratory tests which will be available within the next 2 hours, including a chest x ray, electrocardiogram, urinalysis, blood counts, glucose, BUN, and electrolytes which may disclose anemia, infection, diabetes, uremia, polymyalgia rheumatica, hyponatremia and hypokalemia, all of which are common causes of "weakness." (Testing for serum phosphate and calcium are also valuable if available.)
- If no etiology for weakness can be found, probe the patient, family, and friends once again for any hidden agenda, and if none is found, reassure them about all the serious illnesses which have been ruled out. At this time, discharge the patient and make arrangements for definite followup.

What not to do:

- Do not order any laboratory tests the results of which you will not see. Your best strategy is to stick to tests which will return while the patient is in the emergency department, and defer any long investigations to the followup physician. Laboratory results which are never seen or acted upon are worse than none at all.
- Do not insist upon making the diagnosis in the emergency department in every case. In this clinical situation, your role in the ED is to rule out acutely life-threatening conditions, and then make arrangements for further evaluations elsewhere.

Discussion

Approach the patient with "weakness" with an open mind and be prepared to take some time with the evaluation. Demonstrable localized weakness usually points to a specific neuromuscular etiology, while generalized weakness is the presenting complaint for a multitude of ills. In young patients, weakness may be a sign of psychological depression while in older patients it may be depression, or also the first sign of a subdural hematoma, pneumonia, urinary tract infection, diabetes, heart failure, or cancer.

It is very important to exclude Guillain-Barré Syndrome as one of the critical, life-threatening etiologies to weakness. The pattern is not always an ascending paralysis or weakness. If the diagnosis is suspected, the patient needs a lumbar puncture. Nerve conduction studies might be helpful, if they could be obtained on an emergency basis. Botulism is another condition that must be excluded by history or observation. Patients who are suffering from muscle weakness, such as in myasthenia gravis or Guillain-Barré Syndrome, get into trouble because they can't breathe. Pulmonary function studies, e.g., vital capacity, are very helpful in selecting patients who might be close to severe respiratory embarrassment.

Vertigo ("Dizzy, lightheaded")

Presentation:

This may be a nonspecific complaint which must be refined further into an altered somatic sensation (giddiness, wooziness); orthostatic changes (lightheadedness, fainting); fear of heights or acrophobia ("vertigo" of popular fiction); or the sensation of the environment (or patient) spinning (true vertigo). True vertigo is virtually always accompanied by nystagmus, which is the ocular compensation for the unreal sensation of spinning; but the nystagmus may be extinguished when the eyes are open and fixed on some point (by the same token, vertigo is usually worse with the eyes closed). Nausea and vomiting are common accompanying symptoms, along with (depending on the underlying cause) hearing changes, tinnitus, cerebellar or adjacent cranial nerve impairment.

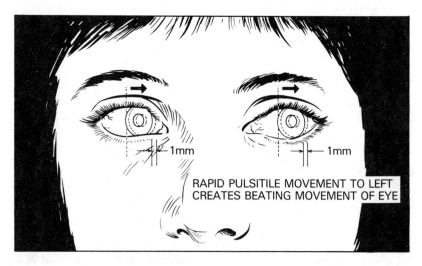

1mm

1mm

RAPID PULSITILE MOVEMENT TO LEFT
CREATES BEATING MOVEMENT OF EYE

What to do:

- Ask specifically about the sensation of spinning, factors which make it better or worse, and associated symptoms. Ask about drugs or toxins which could be responsible.
- Examine for nystagmus, which can be horizontal, vertical or rotatory (pupils describe arcs). You may bring out nystagmus on extremes of gaze. If it is horizontal, bring the inner edge of the contralateral iris even with the inner canthus, and watch whether there are more than the normal 2 to 3 beats of nystagmus before the eyes are still. You may detect nystagmus when the eyes are closed by watching the bulge of the cornea moving under the lid.
- If nystagmus is not clearly evident and the patient can tolerate it, attempt a provocative mancuver for positional nystagmus by having the patient rapidly sit up and then lie back, hanging his head over the edge of the stretcher and turning his head and moving his eyes from side to side.
- Examine ears for cerumen, foreign bodies, otitis media, and hearing.
- Examine all the cranial nerves. Test cerebellar function (rapid alternating movement, finger-nose, gait).

  There is a need to check the corneal reflexes. If absent on one side in a patient who does not wear contact lenses, consider acoustic neuroma.

- Decide, on the basis of the above, whether the etiology is central (brainstem, cerebellopontine angle tumor, multiple sclerosis) or peripheral (vestibular organs, eighth nerve). Central lesions may require further workup, otolaryngologic or neurologic consultation, or hospital admission, while peripheral lesions, although more symptomatic, are more likely self-limiting.
- Treat vertigo symptoms with diazepam (Valium) 5–10mg qid, meclizine (Antivert) 12.5–25mg qid, hydroxyzine (Vistaril) 25mg qid, or promethazine (Phenergan) 25mg qid, and bedrest as needed until symptoms improve. The first dose may be given in the emergency department. If the patient does not respond, he may require hospitalization for further parenteral treatment.
- Arrange for followup if there is no clear improvement in 2 days.

What not to do:

Do not make the diagnosis of Ménière's disease (endolymphatic hydrops) without the triad of paroxysmal vertigo, sensorineural deafness, and tinnitus.

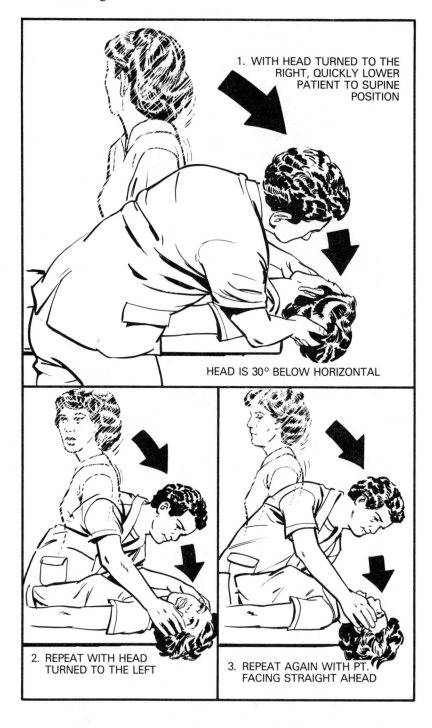

Discussion:

Peripheral etiologies of vertigo/nystagmus tend to be irritation of the ear (utricle, saccule, semicircular canals) or the vestibular division of the eighth cranial (acoustic) nerve by toxins otitis, viral infection, or cerumen or a foreign body against the tympanic membrane. The term "labyrinthitis" should be reserved for vertigo with hearing changes, and "vestibular neuronitis" for the common short-lived vertigo without hearing changes usually associated with viral upper respiratory infections. "Benign positional nystagmus" is fairly common in older patients with cervical spondylosis, but, as it tends to be chronic and might be associated with vertebrobasilar insufficiency, a suggestion of this diagnosis still merits a neurologic followup. "Benign paroxysmal positional vertigo" may strike at any age, and may be related to dislocated otoconia in the utricle and saccule. If it occurs following trauma, suspect a basal skull fracture with leakage of endolymph or perilymph.

Central etiologies include vertebrobasilar arterial insufficiency (associated symptoms are nausea, vomiting, ataxia, cranial nerve, or cerebellar signs), multiple sclerosis, temporal lobe epilepsy, basilar migraine, and tumors of the cerebellopontine angle (e.g., acoustic neuromas, the earliest sign of which is usually a gradual loss of auditory discrimination; and posterior fossa tumors, which may produce cerebellar ataxia).

Either central or peripheral nystagmus can be due to toxins, most commonly alcohol, tobacco, aminoglycosides, minocycline, disopyramide, phencyclidine, and carbon monoxide. Vertigo can also be part of an allergic reaction, usually to shellfish.

Transdermal scopolamine has been useful for prophylaxis of motion sickness, and may be an effective treatment for vertigo as well.

Vertigo

Classification of Nystagmus

	Central	*Peripheral*
History	insidious onset continuous for months	sudden onset intermittent brief episodes
Symptoms	few or none	vertigo corresponds with nystagmus
Hearing changes	none	tinnitus, unilateral deafness
Associated findings	cerebellar ataxia other cranial nerve abnormalities	nausea, vomiting only VIII involved
Direction of spontaneous nystagmus	vertical, horizontal	rotatory, horizontal
Positional nystagmus	immediate onset does not fatigue with repetition few symptoms	nystagmus lags 3–10 sec behind change in position, lasts about 10 sec less nystagmus when maneuver repeated
Site affected	brainstem, cerebellum	labyrinth, acoustic nerve (VIII)
Diagnosis	vertebrobasilar TIA acoustic neuroma posterior fossa tumor multiple sclerosis basilar migraine temporal lobe epilepsy toxic	otitis vestibular neuronitis labyrinthitis benign positional nystagmus benign paroxysmal positional nystagmus Ménière's cerumen, FB toxic

Bell's Palsy (Facial Weakness)

Presentation:

An adult complains of sudden onset of "numbness," a feeling of fullness or swelling, pain or some other change in sensation on one side of the face; a crooked smile, mouth "drawing" or some other asymmetrical weakness of facial muscles; an irritated, dry or tearing eye; drooling out of the corner of the mouth; or changes in hearing or taste. Often there will have been a viral illness one to three weeks before.

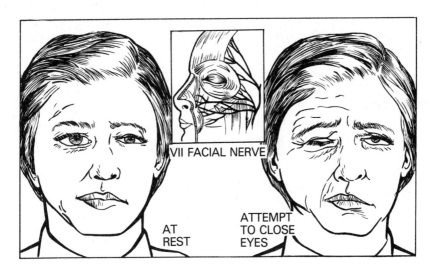

VII FACIAL NERVE

AT REST   ATTEMPT TO CLOSE EYES

What to do:

- Perform a thorough neurological examination of cranial and upper cervical nerves, and limb strength, noting which are involved, and whether unilaterally or bilaterally. Check tearing, corneal dessication, hearing, and, when practical, taste. Examine the ear canals for herpetic vesicles and the tympanic membrane for signs of otitis media.
- If the cornea is dry or injured from the patient's inability to make tears and blink, protect it by patching (see "Corneal Abrasion").
- If the diagnosis is clearly an early idiopathic cranial nerve palsy, (Bell's palsy) not caused or complicated by trauma, infection, or diabetes, try to ameliorate symptons with a short course of corticosteroids (e.g., prednisone 60mg qd for 10 days).

- Reassure the patient that 80–90% of cases of Bell's palsy recover completely in a few weeks, but provide for definite followup and reevaluation.

What not to do:

- Do not forget alternate causes of facial palsy which require different treatment, such as cerebrovascular accidents and cerebellopontine angle tumors (which usually produce weakness in limbs or defects of adjacent cranial nerves), multiple sclerosis (which is usually not painful, spares taste, and often produces intranuclear ophthalmoplegia), Ramsay Hunt syndrome (or herpes zoster of the geniculate ganglion, which causes decreased hearing, pain, and vesicles in the ear canal), and polio (which presents as fever, headache, neck stiffness, and palsies).

Discussion:

Although Bell's palsy was described classically as a pure facial nerve lesion, and physicians have tried to identify the exact level at which the nerve is compressed, the most common presenting complaints of patients are related to trigeminal nerve involvement. The mechanism is probably a spotty demyelination of several nerves at several sites, caused by a viral infection.

2

Ophthalmologic

Periorbital Ecchymosis (Black Eye)

Presentation:

The patient has been struck about the eye, most often with a fist, and is alarmed because of the swelling and discoloration. There may be an associated subconjunctival hemorrhage, but the remainder of the eye exam should be negative and there should be no palpable bony deformities.

What to do:

- Clarify as well as possible the specific mechanism of injury. A fist is much less likely to cause serious injury than a baseball bat.
- Perform a complete eye exam including a bright light exam to rule out an early hyphema, a funduscopic exam to rule out a retinal detachment or dislocated lens, and a fluorescein stain to rule out a corneal abrasion. Visual acuity testing should always be performed.

  Special attention should be given to ruling out a blow-out fracture of the orbital floor or wall. Test extraocular eye movements, especially upward gaze, and check sensation over the infraorbital nerve distribution. Enophthalmus is usually not observed, although it is part of the classic textbook triad associated with a blow-out fracture.
- Symmetrically palpate the supra- and infraorbital rims as well as the zygoma, feeling for a deformity such as one would encounter with a displaced tripod fracture. A unilateral deformity will be obvious if your thumbs are fixed in a midline position while you use your index fingers to palpate the patient's facial bones simultaneously both left and right.

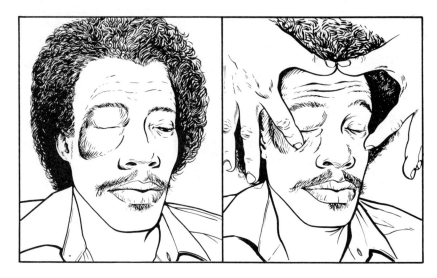

- When there is a substantial mechanism of injury or if there is any clinical suspicion of an underlying fracture, obtain x rays of the orbit.
- When a significant injury has been ruled out, reassure the patient that there is no serious problem. The swelling will subside within 12–24 hrs with use of a cold pack and the discoloration will take approximately a week to 10 days to clear. Acetaminophen should be all that is required for analgesia.

What not to do:

- Do not brush off the patient's problem as a minor annoyance. This is an emotionally upsetting injury and the patient needs a sympathetic approach if he is to be satisfied with his care.
- Do not use proteolytic enzymes. They do no significant good and they may do significant harm.
- Do not get unnecessary radiographs. Minor injuries with normal eye exams and no palpable deformities do not require x rays.
- Do not brush off bilateral deep periorbital ecchymoses ("raccoon eyes") especially if caused by head trauma remote to the eye. This may be the only sign of a basilar skull fracture.

Discussion:

Black eyes are most commonly nothing more than uncomplicated facial contusions. Patients become upset about them because they are so "near the eye," because they produce such noticeable facial disfigurement, and because there is often secondary gain being sought against the person who hit them. Nonetheless, serious injury must always be considered and ruled out prior to the patient's discharge from your care.

Conjunctivitis

Presentation:

The patient will complain of a red eye, a sensation of fullness, burning, itching, or scratching, and perhaps a foreign body sensation and tearing. Examination will disclose generalized infection of the conjunctiva, thinning out towards the cornea (localized inflammation suggests some other diagnosis such as a foreign body, episcleritis, or a viral or bacterial ulcer). Pain, photophobia, and a limbal blush suggest involvement of the cornea and iris.

Different symptoms suggest different etiologies. Tearing, lymphadenopathy, and upper respiratory symptoms suggest a viral conjunctivitis; pain upon awakening and a copious purulent exudate suggests a bacterial conjunctivitis; few symptoms upon awakening but discomfort worsening during the day suggests a dry eye; and a seasonal recurrence of chemosis and itching, with cobblestone hypertrophy of the tarsal conjunctiva, suggests allergic, or vernal, conjunctivitis.

What to do:

- Examine the eye, including visual acuity, inspection for foreign bodies, pupillary reaction fundoscopy, estimation of intraocular pressure by palpation of the globe above the tarsal plate, slit lamp examination (when available), and fluorescein and ultraviolet blue light to assess the corneal epithelium.
- Ask about and look for any rash, arthritis, or mucous membrane involvement which could point to Stevens-Johnson syndrome, Kawasaki's, Reiter's, or some other ailment that can present with conjunctivitis.
- If the diagnosis is viral or bacterial conjunctivitis, start the patient on warm compresses and topical antibiotic ophthalmic ointment (which transiently blurs vision (e.g., erythromycin, sulfa, or gentamycin) every 4 hours, or antibiotic solution (which does not affect vision (e.g., 10% sulfacetamide) every hour.
- For allergic conjunctivitis, use cold compresses and weak top-

ical vasoconstrictors (e.g., Vasocon-A) unless the patient has a shallow anterior chamber that would be prone to acute angle-closure glaucoma (see p 34).

- If the problem is dry eyes, or keratoconjunctivitis sicca, use methylcellulose (Dacriose) artificial tear drops.
- Have the patient followup with the ophthalmologist if the infection does not clearly resolve in 2 days, or if there is any involvement of cornea or iris.

What not to do:

- Do not forget to wash your hands and equipment after examining the patient, or you may spread herpes simplex or epidemic keratoconjunctivitis to yourself and other patients.
- Do not patch an affected eye, as this interferes with the cleansing function of tear flow.

Discussion:

Most viral and bacterial conjunctivitis will resolve spontaneously, with the possible exception of staphylococcus, meningiococcus, and gonococcus infections, which can produce destructive sequelae without treatment. Routine conjunctival cultures are seldom of much value, but you probably should Gram stain or culture a really copious purulent exudate. Although they may not always be necessary, antibiotic ointments or drops and warm compresses are quite soothing for the patient. Neomycin-containing ointments should probably be avoided, because allergic sensitization to this antibiotic is common. Any corneal ulceration requires ophthalmological consultation.

Iritis

Presentation:

The patient usually complains of eye pain, blurred vision, and photophobia. He may have had a pink eye for a few days, trauma during the previous day, or no overt previous eye problem.

When you look through any accompanying conjunctivitis to the junction of the cornea and conjunctiva (the limbus) you will see a pink blush which, on close inspection, is a tangle of fine cilliary vessels, visible through the white sclera. This limbal blush is usually the earliest sign of iritis; it may require a slit lamp or other magnification to be seen.

As the iritis becomes more pronounced, the iris and ciliary muscles go into spasm, producing an irregular and constricted pupil and a lens which will not focus. The slit lamp may demonstrate white blood cells or light reflection from a protein exudate in the clear aqueous humor of the anterior chamber.

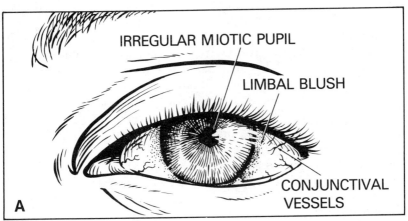

IRREGULAR MIOTIC PUPIL

LIMBAL BLUSH

CONJUNCTIVAL VESSELS

A

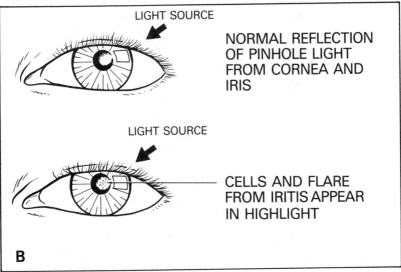

LIGHT SOURCE

NORMAL REFLECTION OF PINHOLE LIGHT FROM CORNEA AND IRIS

LIGHT SOURCE

CELLS AND FLARE FROM IRITIS APPEAR IN HIGHLIGHT

B

What to do:

- Perform a complete eye exam, including topical anesthesia if necessary for the exam; visual acuity, pupillary reflexes and accommodation; funduscopy; slit lamp examination of the anterior chamber, including pinhole illumination to bring out cells and flare; and fluorescein for the cornea.

- Attempt to ascertain the cause of the iritis (is it generalized from a corneal insult or conjunctivitis, a late sequela of blunt trauma, infectious, or autoimmune?)
- Explain to the patient the potential severity of the problem—this is no routine conjunctivitis, but a process which can develop into blindness.
- Arrange for ophthalmologic consultation or followup, and, if acceptable to the consulting ophthalmologist . . .
- Dilate the pupil and paralyze ciliary accommodation [e.g., with 1% cyclopentolate (Cyclogyl) drops once], which will not only relieve the pain of the muscle spasm, but will keep the iris away from the lens, where meiosis and inflammation might cause adhesions (posterior synechiae). For a prolonged effect, instill 1 drop of Homatropine 5% before discharge.
- Suppress the inflammation with topical steroids [e.g., 1% prednisolone (Inflamase) drops once];
- Prescribe po pain medicine if needed; and
- Double check that the patient is seen the next day in followup.

What not to do:

- Do not let the patient shrug off his "pink eye" and escape followup, even if he is feeling better, because of the real possibility of permanent visual impairment.
- Do not overlook a penetrating foreign body as the cause of the inflammation.
- Avoid dilating an eye with a shallow anterior chamber and precipitating acute angle closure glaucoma.

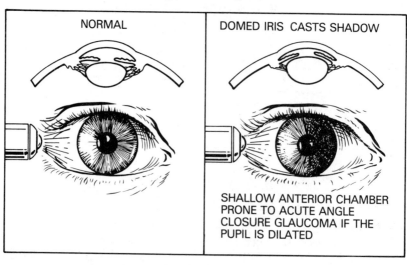

NORMAL

DOMED IRIS CASTS SHADOW

SHALLOW ANTERIOR CHAMBER PRONE TO ACUTE ANGLE CLOSURE GLAUCOMA IF THE PUPIL IS DILATED

Discussion:

Iritis (or anterior uveitis) may be caused by many ailments, but always represents a real threat to vision which requires emergency treatment and expert followup. The inflammatory process in the anterior eye can opacify the anterior chamber, deform the iris or lens, scar them together, or extend into adjacent structures. Posterior synechiae can potentiate cataracts and glaucoma. Treatment with topical steroids can backfire if the process is caused by an infection (especially herpes keratitis); thus the slit lamp examination is especially useful.

Sometimes an intense conjunctivitis or keratitis may produce some sympathetic limbal blush, which will resolve as the primary process resolves, and require no additional treatment. A more definite, but still mild, iritis, may resolve with cycloplegics, and not require steroids. All of these, however, mandate ophthalmologic consultation and followup.

Conjunctival Foreign Body

Presentation:

Low-velocity projectiles, like wind blown dust particles, can be loose in the tear film or lodged in a conjunctival sac. The patient may not be very accurate in locating the foreign body by sensation alone.

On exam, normally occurring white papules inside lids can be mistaken for foreign bodies, and transparent foreign bodies can be invisible in the tear film (until outlined by fluorescein).

What to do:

- Instill topical anesthetic drops.
- Perform visual acuity and funduscopy, bright light the anterior chamber and tear film (best done with a slit lamp) and examine the conjunctival sacs.

    To examine the lower sac, pull the lower lid down with your finger while the patient looks up.

    To examine the upper sac, hold the base of the upper lid down with a cotton-tipped swab while pulling the lid out and up by its lashes, everting most of the lid, as the patient looks down. Push the cotton swab downward to help turn the upper conjunctival sac "inside out." The stiff tarsal plate usually keeps the upper lid everted after the swab is removed, and as long as the patient continues looking down. Looking up reduces the lid to its usual position.

- A loose foreign body may adhere to a swab lightly touched to the surface of the eye, or be washed out by copious irrigation with saline.
- Perform a fluorescein exam to disclose any corneal abrasion caused by the foreign body. These vertical scratches occur when the lid blinks over a coarse object and should be treated as described on p 40.
- Follow with saline irrigation for possible fragments.

What not to do:

- Do not overlook a foreign body in the deep recesses of the upper conjunctival sac.
- Do not overlook an embedded or penetrating foreign body.
- Do not overlook a corneal abrasion.

Discussion:

Good first aid (copious irrigation and not rubbing eyes) will take care of most ocular foreign bodies. The history of injury with a high-velocity fragment such as a metal shard chipped off a hammer or chisel, should raise the question of a penetrating foreign body and special x rays should be obtained. Techniques for conjunctival foreign body removal can also be applied to locating a displaced contact lens, (p 49) but be aware that fluorescein dye absorbed by soft contact lenses fades slowly.

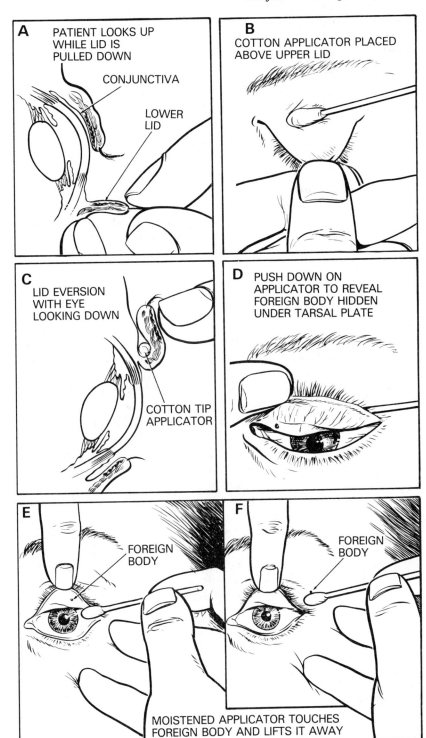

A — PATIENT LOOKS UP WHILE LID IS PULLED DOWN
CONJUNCTIVA
LOWER LID

B — COTTON APPLICATOR PLACED ABOVE UPPER LID

C — LID EVERSION WITH EYE LOOKING DOWN
COTTON TIP APPLICATOR

D — PUSH DOWN ON APPLICATOR TO REVEAL FOREIGN BODY HIDDEN UNDER TARSAL PLATE

E — FOREIGN BODY

F — FOREIGN BODY

MOISTENED APPLICATOR TOUCHES FOREIGN BODY AND LIFTS IT AWAY

Corneal Foreign Body

Presentation:

The eye has been struck by a falling or blowing fragment, or a loose foreign body has become embedded by rubbing, thereby producing intense pain. Moderate-to-high-velocity foreign bodies (e.g., fragments chipped off a chisel by a hammer or spray from a grinding wheel) can be superficially embedded or lodged deep in the vitreous.

Superficial foreign bodies may be visible during simple side-lighting of the cornea or by slit lamp examination. Deep foreign bodies may be visible only as moving shadows on funduscopy, with a trivial-appearing or invisible puncture in the sclera.

What to do:

- Instill topical anesthetic drops.
- Perform visual acuity and funduscopy (look for shadows), bright light anterior chamber (slit lamp is best), and check pupillary reflexes (for iritis) and conjunctivae (for loose foreign bodies).
- A barely embedded foreign body might be touched out with a moistened swab as shown in the section on the conjunctival foreign body, but if firmly embedded, it will have to be scooped out (under magnification) with an ophthalmic spud or an 18-gauge needle. Give the patient an object to fixate upon to keep his eye still, brace your hand on his forehead or cheek, and approach the eye tangentially so no sudden motion can cause a perforation of the anterior chamber. Removal of the foreign body leaves a defect which is treated as a corneal abrasion. If a rust ring is present, it will appear that a foreign body remains adherent to the cornea. Use the needle to continue to scrape away this rust-impregnated corneal epithelium. A corneal burr is very effective and safe for this task.

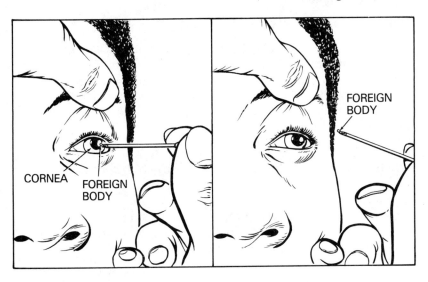

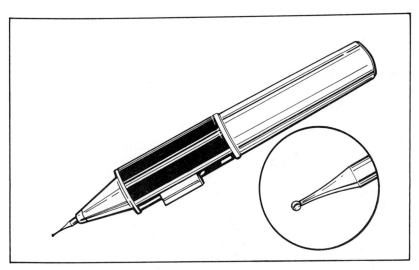

- If unclear, perform a fluorescein exam to document the extent of the corneal defect.
- Finish with further irrigation for possible fragments, antibiotic ointment, eye patch, and anti-inflammatory medication (Percodan, aspirin, etc.), the first dose given before leaving the ED.
- Make an appointment for ophthalmologic followup the next day, to evaluate healing and any residual foreign bodies.

What not to do:

- Do not overlook a foreign body deep inside the globe—the delayed inflammatory response can lead to blindness.
- Do not leave an iron foreign body in place without arranging early ophthalmic followup.

Discussion:

Decide beforehand how much time you will spend (and how much trauma you will inflict on the cornea) before giving up on removing a corneal foreign body and calling your ophthalmologic consultant.

Some ED physicians recommend using a small needle for scooping, to minimize the possibility of a corneal perforation, but with a tangential approach the larger needle is better.

Corneal Abrasion

Presentation:

The patient will usually complain of severe eye pain following eye trauma or a foreign body, but a corneal abrasion can occur without identifiable trauma, or following prolonged wearing of a hard contact lens.

Often the patient cannot open his eye for the exam. Abrasions are occasionally visible on sidelighting the cornea. (Conjunctival inflammation can range from nothing to severe conjunctivitis with accompanying iritis.)

What to do:

- Instill topical anesthetic drops (to permit exam).
- Perform a complete eye exam (visual acuity, funduscopy, anterior chamber bright light, conjunctival sacs).
- Perform the fluorescein exam by wetting a paper strip impregnated with dry orange fluorescein dye and touching this strip into the tear pool inside the lower conjunctival sac. After the patient blinks, darken the room and examine the patient's eye under blue or ultraviolet light (the red-free light on the ophthalmoscope does not work). Areas of denuded or devitalized corneal epithelium will fluoresce green.

- If a foreign body is present, remove it and irrigate the eye.
- If iritis is present (evidenced by photophobia, an irregular pupil or meiosis, and a limbic blush in addition to conjunctival injection) consult the ophthalmologic followup physician about starting the patient on topical mydriatics and steroids (e.g., Cyclogyl and Inflamase).
- After instilling antibiotic ointment, patch the eye with enough pressure to keep the lid closed by folding one eyepatch double to rest against the lid, covering it with a second eyepatch, and taping both tightly with several strips of 1″ tape running from the cheek to mid-forehead.

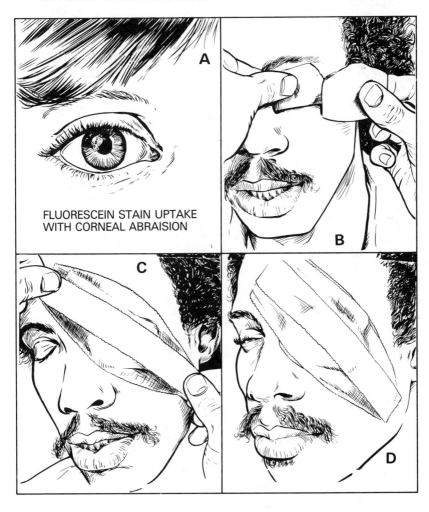

FLUORESCEIN STAIN UPTAKE WITH CORNEAL ABRAISION

- Prescribe anti-inflammatory analgesics (Percodan, Empirin with codeine, Motrin, aspirin, etc.), and give the first dose in the ED.
- Tell the patient the pain will return when the local anesthetic wears off.
- Make an appointment for ophthalmologic followup to remove the dressing and reevaluate the abrasion the next day.

What not to do:

- Do not give patient any topical anesthetic for continued instillation.

Discussion:

Fluorescein binds to corneal stroma and devitalized epithelium, but not to intact corneal epithelium. Collections of fluorescein elsewhere, in conjunctival irregularities and in the tear film, are not pathological.

Hard contact lenses can abrade the cornea, but can also cause diffuse ischemic damage when worn for more than 12 hours at a time, by depriving the avascular corneal epithelium of oxygen and nutrients in the tear layer.

Continuous instillation of topical anesthetic drops can impair healing, inhibit protective reflexes, permit further eye injury, and even cause sloughing of the corneal epithelium.

Periorbital and Conjunctival Edema

Presentation:

The patient is frightened by the facial distortion and itching that seem to appear spontaneously or up to 24 hours after having been bitten by a bug or having contacted some irritant. There may be minimal to marked generalized conjunctival swelling (chemosis), but little injection. Tenderness should be minimal or absent and there should be no fever. The patient may have been rubbing his eye—in fact, an allergen or chemical irritant on the hand may cause periorbital edema long before a reaction, if any, is evident on the skin of the hand.

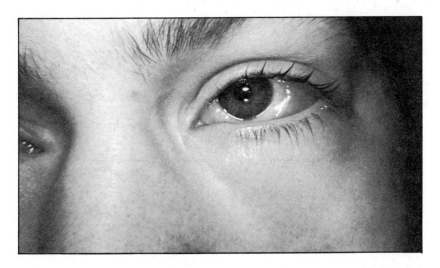

What to do:

- After completing a full eye exam, reassure the patient that this is not as serious as it looks.
- Prescribe hydroxyzine (Atarax) 50mg q6h for mild to moderate swelling and a six-day course of steroids (e.g., Aristopak 4mg) for more severe cases. Vasocon-A Ophthalmic drops will be soothing and reduce swelling when the conjunctiva is involved.
- Instruct the patient to use cool compresses to reduce swelling and discomfort.
- Inquire about the cause, including allergies and chemical irritants.
- Warn the patient about the potential signs of infection.

What not to do:

- Do not confuse this with periorbital cellulitis (pain, heat, fever, deep erythema). Periorbital cellulitis requires hospitalization and aggressive antibiotic therapy.
- Do not apply heat—swelling and pruritis will increase.

Discussion:

The dramatic swelling that often brings a patient to an emergency department occurs because of the loose connective tissue surrounding the orbit. Fluid quickly accumulates when a local allergic response causes increased capillary permeability, resulting in dramatic eyelid swelling. The envenomation, allergen, or irritant responsible may actually be located some distance away on the face (or hand) but the loose periorbital tissue is the first to swell.

Subconjunctival Hemorrhage

Presentation:

This condition may be spontaneous or follow a minor trauma, coughing episode, vomiting, or drinking binge. There is no pain or visual loss, but the patient may be frightened by the appearance of his eye and have some sensation of superficial fullness.

This hemorrhage usually appears as a bright red area covering part of the sclera, but contained by conjunctiva. It may cover the whole visible globe, sparing only the cornea.

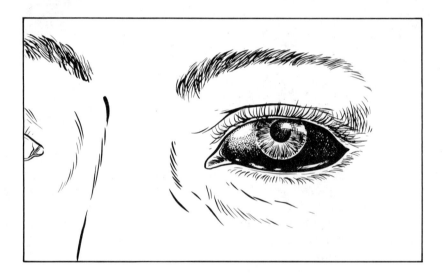

What to do:

- Look for associated trauma, or other signs of a potential bleeding disorder.
- Perform a complete eye exam that includes:
  a) Visual acuity testing
  b) Inspection of conjunctival sacs
  c) Bright lighting the anterior chamber
  d) Testing extraocular movements
  e) Fluorescein staining and funduscopic examination
- Reassure the patient that there is no serious eye damage—explain that the blood may continue to spread, but that all the redness should resolve in about 5–7 days.

What not to do:

- Don't forget to tell the patient that the redness may spread.
- Don't ignore any significant finding discovered on the complete eye exam.

Discussion:

Success at reassuring the patient will best be accomplished by openly recognizing the patient's fear in a compassionate manner, performing a complete eye exam before informing the patient that, although this looks serious, it is only a harmless, broken blood vessel.

Ultraviolet Keratoconjunctivitis ("Welder's Burn")

Presentation:

The patient arrives with burning eye pain, usually bilateral, beginning 6 to 8 hours after a brief exposure to a high intensity ultraviolet light source such as a sunlamp or welder's arc. The eye exam shows conjunctival injection; fluorescein staining shows diffuse superficial uptake (discerned as a punctate keratopathy under slitlamp examination). The patient may also have first-degree skin burns.

What to do:

- Apply topical anesthetic ophthalmic drops (once, to permit exam).
- Perform a complete eye exam (visual acuity, funduscopic, anterior chamber bright light, fluorescein, inspection of conjunctival sacs).
- Instill an antibiotic ointment and patch eyes for approximately 12 hours. Cold compresses, rest, and anti-inflammatory analgesics (e.g., Percodan, Motrin, aspirin with codeine) should be prescribed to control pain. The first dose can be given in the ED. If the pain is severe, giving the patient a sleeping pill would be helpful.
- Warn the patient that pain will return when the local anesthetic wears off, but that the pills prescribed should help to relieve it.

What not to do:

- Do not give the patient a topical anesthetic for continued instillation. It can slow healing and increases the risk of eye injury.

Discussion:

The history of a brief exposure may be difficult to elicit after the long asymptomatic interval. Longer exposures to lower intensity UV sources may resemble a sunburn.

Some physicians find it quite acceptable to substitute for the antibiotic ointment a one-time instillation of an ophthalmic anesthetic ointment (Tetracaine), which allows longer-lasting topical anesthesia.

Hordeolum (Sty)

Presentation:

The patient complains of redness, swelling, and pain in the eye or eyelid, perhaps at the base of an eyelash (sty or external hordeolum) or deep within the lid (meibomianitis or internal hordeolum, best appreciated with the lid everted) perhaps with conjunctivitis and purulent drainage.

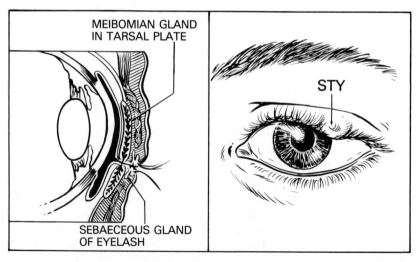

MEIBOMIAN GLAND
IN TARSAL PLATE

STY

SEBAECEOUS GLAND
OF EYELASH

What to do:

- Examine the eye, including visual acuity and inversion of lids (see "Conjunctival FB" for technique).
- Show patient how to instill antibiotic drops or ointment (e.g., sulfa, erythromycin, gentamycin) into his lower conjunctival sac and apply warm compresses for 10 minutes per hour.
- Instruct the patient to return to the ophthalmologist or the ED if the problem is not clearly resolving in two days, or if it gets any worse.
- If the abscess does not spontaneously drain or resolve in two days, you may incise it with the tip of a #11 blade or small needle, with the same followup instructions.

What not to do:

- Do not miss a periorbital cellulitis, which requires systemic antibiotic treatment.

Discussion:

The terminology of the two types of hordeolum have become confusing. Meibomian glands run vertically, within the tarsal plate, open at tiny puncta along the lid margin, and secrete oil to coat the tear film. The glands of Zeiss and Moll are the sebaceous glands opening into the follicles of the eyelashes. Both can become occluded and superinfected, producing meibomianitis (internal hordeolum) or a sty (external hordeolum). The ED care of both acute infections is the same. A chronic granuloma of the meibomian gland is called a chalazion, will not drain, and requires excision.

Contact Lens Overwear

Presentation:

A patient who wears hard contact lenses comes to the ED in the early morning complaining of severe eye pain. He has fallen asleep with his lenses in or stayed up late, leaving his lenses in for more than 12 hours.

He may not be able to open his eyes for examination because of pain and blepharospasm. He may show obvious corneal injury, with signs of iritis and conjunctivitis, or show no visible findings at all without fluorescein staining. This staining should demonstrate central corneal uptake of fluorescein without sharply demarcated borders.

What to do:

- Instill topical anesthestic drops.
- Perform a complete eye exam including pupillary reflexes, funduscopy, and inspection of conjunctival sacs.
- Instill fluorescein dye (use single-dose dropper or wet a dye-impregnated paper strip and touch it to the tear pool in the lower conjunctival sac), have the patient blink, and examine under blue or ultraviolet light for the green fluorescence of dye bound to devitalized corneal epithelium.

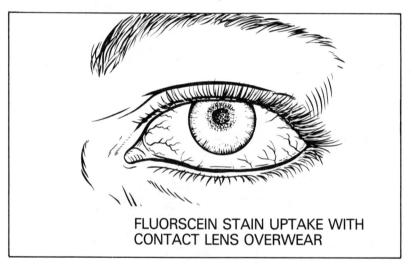

FLUORSCEIN STAIN UPTAKE WITH
CONTACT LENS OVERWEAR

- Sketch the area of corneal injury on the patient record, rinse out the dye, instill antibiotic ointment in the lower conjunctival sac, and patch the eye as shown in "Corneal Abrasion."
- Prescribe anti-inflammatory analgesics (e.g., aspirin, Motrin, Percodan) and give the first dose in the ED.
- Instruct the patient to avoid wearing his lenses for 4–5 days, and to seek ophthalmologic followup within one day.

What not to do:

- Do not discharge a patient with topical anesthetic ophthalmic drops for continued administration; they not only potentiate further injury, but also impair healing.
- Do not discharge an unaccompanied patient with both eyes patched.

Discussion:

Hard contact lenses left in place too long deprive the avascular corneal epithelium of oxygen and nutrients from the tear film. This produces diffuse ischemia, which usually heals perfectly in a day, but can be exquisitely painful as soon as the lenses are removed.

Removal of Dislocated Contact Lens

Presentation:

The patient may know the lens has dislocated into one of the recesses of the conjunctiva, and complain only of the loss of refractory correction; or he may have lost track of the lens completely, in which case the eye is a logical place to look first. Pain and blepharospasm suggest a corneal abrasion, perhaps from removal attempts.

What to do:

- If pain and blepharospasm are a problem, topically anesthetize the eye.
- Pull back lids as when looking for conjunctival foreign bodies, invert the upper lid, and, if necessary instill fluorescein dye *(a last resort with soft lenses, which absorb the dye tenaciously).*
- If the lens is loose, slide it over the cornea, and let the patient remove it in the usual manner. Irrigation may loosen a dry, stuck lens.
- For a more adherent hard lens, use a commercially available suction cup lens remover. Soft lenses may be pinched between fingers or require a commercially available rubber pincer.
- Put the lens in a proper container (sterile saline is always right).
- Complete the eye examination, including acuity, slit lamp and fluorescein examination. Patch the eye if there is a corneal abrasion.
- Instruct the patient not to wear the lens until all symptoms have abated for 24 hours, and to see his ophthalmologist if there are any problems.

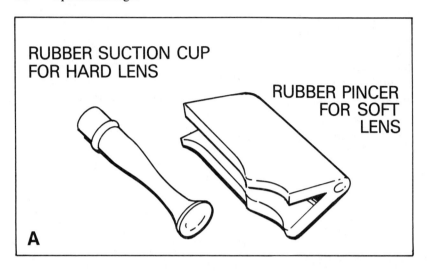

RUBBER SUCTION CUP
FOR HARD LENS

RUBBER PINCER
FOR SOFT
LENS

A

What not to do:

- Do not give up too easily. Lost lenses have been excavated years later from under scar tissue in the conjunctival recesses.
- Don't omit the fluorescein step for fear of spoiling a soft contact lens. The dye may take a long time to elute out, but it is more important to find the dislocated lens.

Discussion:

The deepest recess in the conjunctiva is under the upper lid, but lenses can lodge anywhere; there have been rare cases of lenses perforating the conjunctival sac and migrating posterior to the globe.

Removal of Contact Lens in Unconscious Patient

Presentation:

An unconscious patient, his primary problem under control, is being admitted to the hospital, but remains comatose.

What to do:

- Look for hard contact lenses in place over the cornea by side-lighting the cornea. If lenses are present:
- Place two fingers on the upper and lower lids, and spread them back from the cornea and lens.

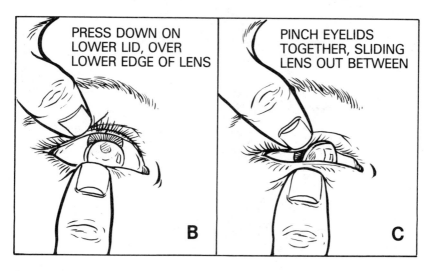

- Slide the edge of the lower lid over the lower edge of the lens and press down gently, causing the upper edge of the lens to tip out.
- Slide the upper lid down until it encounters the upper edge of the lens, and gently pinch the eyelids together, sliding the lens out between them. (If unsuccessful, see techniques on p 49).
- Dress both corneas with antibiotic ointment and tape both eyes shut, to prevent dessication or further injury.
- Put lenses in correct containers (normal saline is always right) labelled "left" and "right."

What not to do:

- Do not bother removing soft or extended wear lenses right away. Unlike hard contact lenses, they are not apt to cause any damage if left in place over the cornea for a few hours.
- Do not confuse types of lenses. Generally, hard lenses do not quite cover the cornea, while soft lenses extend out onto the sclera. Some hard lenses, however, do extend out over the sclera, and should be removed as outlined above.

Discussion:

A hard contact lens in place over the cornea too long deprives the underlying epithelium of oxygen and nutrients it normally obtains by diffusion from the tear film, (see p 44) but can also be displaced and abrade the cornea.

3

Ear/Nose/Throat

Cerumen Impaction (Ear Wax Blockage)

Presentation:

The patient may complain of "wax in the ear," a "stuffed up" or foreign body sensation, itching, decreased hearing, tinnitus, or dizziness.

On physical examination, the dark brown, thick, dry cerumen—perhaps packed down against the ear drum, where it does not occur normally—obscures further visualization of the ear canal.

What to do:

- Explain what you are going to do to the patient. Cover him with a waterproof drape, have him hold a basin below his ear, and tilt the ear slightly over it.
- Fill a 20ml syringe with water at approximately 37°C and fit it with a soft tubing catheter. Aim along the anterior superior wall of the external ear canal (visualize directly) and squirt with all your might.

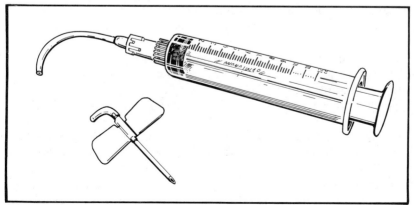

- Repeat until all of the cerumen is gone.
- If multiple attempts at irrigation prove to be unsuccessful, then gentle use of a cerumen spoon (ear curette) may be necessary to pull out the excess wax. Warning the patient about potential discomfort or minor bleeding will save lengthy explanations and apologies later.
- Reexamine the ear and test the patient's hearing.
- Warn the patient that he has thick ear wax, that he may need this procedure done again someday, and that he should never use swabs in his ear.

What not to do:

- Do not irrigate an ear with a suspected or known tympanic membrane perforation, or myringotomy tubes.
- Do not irrigate with a cold (or hot) solution.
- Do not blindly insert a rigid instrument down the canal.

Discussion:

This technique virtually always works within 5–10 squirts. If the irrigation fluid is at body temperature, it will soften the cerumen just enough that it floats out as a plug. If the fluid is too hot or cold it can produce vertigo, nystagmus, nausea, and vomiting.

A conventional blood-drawing syringe, fitted with a butterfly catheter, its tubing cut to 1cm, seems to work better than the big chrome-plated syringes manufactured for irrigating ears. If the external ear canal is not occluded, the risk of perforating the tympanic membrane is infinitesimal. Alternative techniques include adding H_2O_2 to the irrigation fluid (1:1) or using a WaterPik®.

Detergents such as Debrox and Cerumenex are seldom necessary with this technique. They may have some use in prophylaxis, but can also irritate the ear canal.

Cerumen spoons can be dangerous and painful, especially with children, for whom this irrigation technique has proven more effective while providing more reliable assessment of the tympanic membrane.

Cerumen is produced by the sebaceous glands of the hair follicles in the ear canal, and naturally flows outward along these hairs. One of the problems with ear swabs is that they can push wax inwards away from these hairs and against the ear drum, where it can then stick and harden.

Some people have cerumen like oil, while some have cerumen like paraffin, and it is the latter group who are prone to repeated impaction. These people may benefit from use of detergents or glycerin, and occasional irrigation with water, hydrogen peroxide, or acetic acid, but nonetheless, may someday again require your service to "blow out" their ears.

Otitis Externa (Swimmer's Ear)

Presentation:

The patient will complain of ear pain, often accompanied by drainage and a blocked sensation. The pain may be mild or severe and the patient may or may not be febrile. When the condition is mild or chronic there may be itching rather than pain.

Pulling on the auricle or pushing on the tragus of the ear will increase pain.

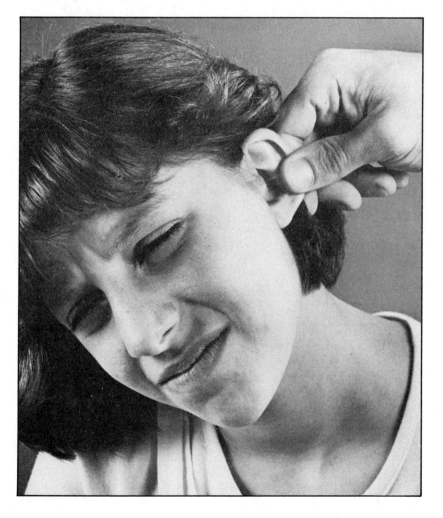

The tissue lining the canal may be swollen and in severe cases the swelling can extend to the soft tissue surrounding the ear. Tender erythematous swelling or an underlying furuncle may be present, and it may be pointing or draining in the outer half of the ear canal. The canal may be erythematous and dry or it may be covered with grayish or black (fungal) plaques. Most often, the canal lining is moist, covered with purulent drainage and debris, and so swollen that it is difficult or impossible to view the tympanic membrane.

What to do:

- Suction out the debris and drainage present in the canal.
- Incise and drain any furuncle that is pointing or fluctuant.
- Insert a narrow gauze wick (cotton or ¼" plain Nugauze) down the length of the canal using a bayonet forceps, or, better, alligator forceps. The Pope ear wick, which expands when wet, may be used as an excellent substitute.

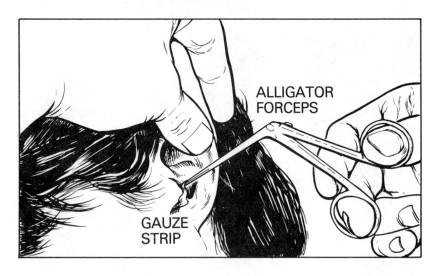

- Prescribe a topical steroid solution for instillation down the wick (e.g., Otic Tridesilon Solution 0.05%), every six to eight hours for the next 7–14 days.
- Have the patient use warm, moist compresses to help relieve any pain or swelling.
- With moderate to severe pain and swelling, prescribe an appropriate analgesic (e.g., acetaminophen, codeine, or oxycodone) and an antibiotic (e.g., dicloxicillin 500mg qid x 10d or cefadroxil 1gm qid x 10d).
- Have the patient use a prophylactic 2% acetic acid solution (e.g., Otic Domeboro Solution) after swimming or bathing when the initial therapy has been completed.

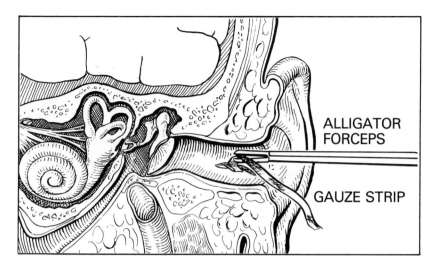

What not to do:

- Do not use neomycin-containing preparations. Neosporin could theoretically cause eighth nerve damage through a perforated TM, and commonly causes contact dermatitis. In addition, long-term use of any topical antibiotics can lead to a fungal superinfection.
- Do not instill medication without first cleansing the ear canal.
- Do not expect medicine to enter a swollen-shut canal without a wick.

Discussion:

Otitis externa has a seasonal occurrence, being more frequently encountered in the summer months, when the climate and contaminated water will most likely precipitate a fungal or bacterial infection. Various dermatoses, diabetes, aggressive ear cleaning with cotton-tipped applicators, and furunculosis also predispose patients to developing otitis externa.

Perforated Tympanic Membrane

Presentation:

The patient will present with ear pain after barotrauma, such as a blow to the ear or deep-water diving; or after direct trauma with a stick or other sharp object. Hemorrhage will often be noticed within the external canal and the patient will experience some hearing loss. Tinnitus or vertigo may also be present. Otoscopic examination will reveal a defect in the tympanic membrane that may or may not be accompanied by disruption of the ossicles.

What to do:

- Clear out any debris from the canal, using gentle suction.
- Test for nystagmus and gross hearing loss.
- Place a protective cotton plug inside of the ear canal and instruct the patient to keep the canal dry.
- Prescribe prophylactic penicillin VK 500mg q6h x 5d.
- Prescribe an appropriate analgesic (e.g., acetaminophen with codeine or oxycodone).
- Insure that the patient gets early followup by an oto-laryngologist.

What not to do:

- Do not instill any fluid into the external canal or allow the patient to get water into his ear. Water in the middle ear is painful, irritating and may introduce bacteria. Covering the cotton plug with petroleum jelly will allow the patient to shower safely.

Discussion:

Small uncomplicated perforations usually heal. When nystagmus, vertigo, profound hearing loss, or disruption of the ossicles is present, then early otolaryngologic consultation is advisable.

Foreign Body—Ear

Presentation:

Sometimes a young child admits to putting something in his ear; sometimes the history is hidden and the child simply presents with a purulent discharge. Most dramatically a patient arrives at the emergency department panic-stricken because he feels and hears a bug crawling around in his ear.

Inspection with an otoscope (suctioning when necessary) reveals the foreign body partially or completely occluding the ear canal. Pebbles, beads, pencil erasers, beans, cotton applicator tips, and tissue paper are common.

What to do:

- If there is a live bug in the patient's ear, simply fill the canal with mineral oil. (Lay the patient on his side and drop the mineral oil down the canal while pulling on the pinna to remove the air bubbles.) This will immediately kill any intruder which can then be removed by using one of the techniques below. The least invasive methods should be attempted first.

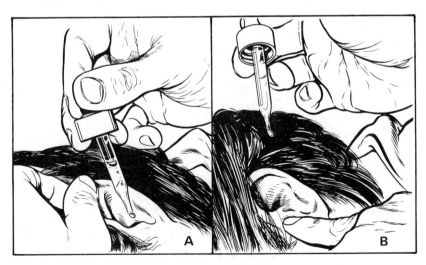

- Water irrigation is often most effective for safely removing a foreign body that is not tightly wedged in the canal. This can be accomplished with an irrigation syringe, WaterPik®, or a standard syringe and cut off scalp vein needle catheter. Tap water or normal saline at body temperature should be used to flush out the foreign body by directing the stream around the object and forcing it out.

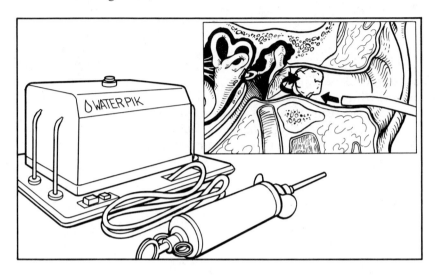

- If irrigation is not successful, attempt to suction out the FB with a standard metal suction tip or specialized flexible tip.

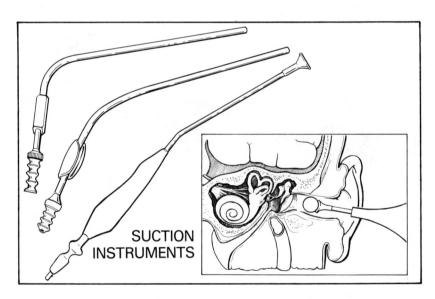

SUCTION INSTRUMENTS

- If the foreign body remains embedded within the canal and your patient is very cooperative, you can attempt to roll or pull the object out using one of the following instruments.

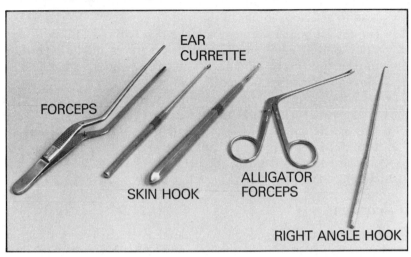

Stabilize the patient's head and fix your hand against it, holding the instrument loosely between your fingers. This will reduce the risk of injury should the patient move suddenly. Under direct visualization through an ear speculum, slide the tip of the instrument behind the foreign body so it can be dragged or rolled out of the ear. Alligator forceps are most useful for removing soft objects like cotton or paper. Simply grab the object between the jaws of the forceps and pull it out.

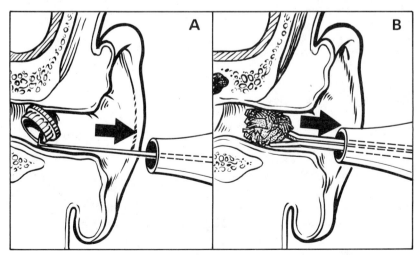

What not to do:

- Do not use a rigid instrument to remove an object from an uncooperative patient's ear. An unexpected movement might lead to a serious injury of the middle ear.
- Do not attempt to remove a large bug without killing it first. They tend to be wily, evasive little creatures and in the heat of battle, the instrument that you are using is very likely to damage the patient's canal.
- Do not attempt to irrigate a tightly wedged bean or seed from an ear canal. The water may cause the bean to swell.
- Do not attempt to remove a large or hard object with bayonet or similar forceps. The bony canal will slowly close the forceps as they are advanced and the object will be pushed farther into the canal.

Discussion:

The cutaneous lining of the bony canal of the ear is very sensitive and is not much affected by topical anesthetics. If your patient is an uncooperative child, the parents should be informed that to reduce risk of serious injury to the eardrum, you are going to have the object removed under general anesthesia by a specialist. Don't make the parents feel guilty because their child is too young to keep still.

Irrigation techniques and the use of the ear curette can also be effective in removing excess cerumen from an ear canal (see p 53). Whenever an instrument is used in an ear canal in an abrasive manner it is a good idea to warn the patient or parents that there may be a small amount of bleeding. Reassurance becomes very difficult after the blood is noted.

Serous Otitis Media

Presentation:

Following an upper respiratory infection or an airplane flight, an adult may complain of a feeling of fullness in the ears, inability to equalize middle ear pressure, decreased hearing, and clicking, popping, or crackling sounds, especially when the head is moved. There is little pain or tenderness.

Through the otoscope the tympanic membrane appears retracted, with a dull to normal light reflex, minimal if any injection, and poor motion on insufflation. You may see an air-fluid level or bubbles through the TM. Hearing will be decreased and the Rinne test will show decreased air conduction (i.e., a tuning fork will be heard no better through air than through bone).

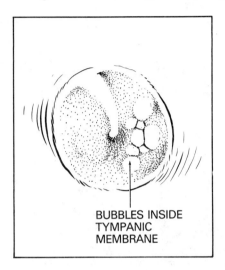

BUBBLES INSIDE
TYMPANIC
MEMBRANE

What to do:

- Tell the patient to lie supine and instill vasoconstrictor nose drops (e.g., phenylephrine [Neo-Synephrine] 1%), wait two minutes for the nasal mucosa to shrink, reinstill nose drops, and wait an additional 2 minutes for the medicine to seep down to the posterior pharyngeal wall, around the opening of the eustachian tube. Have him repeat this procedure with drops (not spray) every 4 hours during the day for no more than 3 days.
- After each treatment with nose drops, instruct the patient to insufflate his middle ear via his eustachian tube by closing his mouth, pinching his nose shut, and blowing until his ears "pop."
- Unless contraindicated by hypertension or other medical conditions, add a systemic vasoconstrictor (e.g., pseudoephedrine 60mg qid).
- Instruct the patient to seek otolaryngologic followup if not better in a week.

What not to do:

- Do not allow the patient to become habituated to vasoconstrictor nose drops. After a few days, they become ineffective, and

then the nasal mucosa develop a rebound swelling known as "rhinitis medicamentosa" when the medicine is withdrawn.
* Do not prescribe antihistamines (which dry out secretions) unless clearly indicated by an allergy.

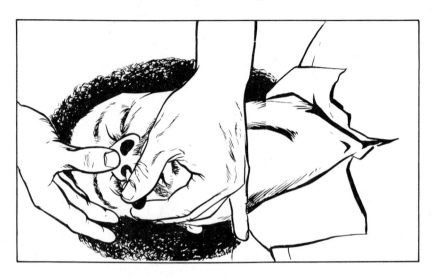

Discussion:

Acute serous otitis media is probably caused by obstruction of the eustachian tube, allowing negative pressure to build up in the middle ear, which then draws a fluid transudate out of the middle ear epithelium. The ED treatment above is directed solely at reestablishing the patency of the eustachian tube, but further treatment includes insufflation of the eustachian tube or myringotomy. Fluid in the middle ear is not only more common in children, because of the underdeveloped eustachian tube, but also more prone to bacterial superinfection, and probably merits prophylactic antibiotics (usually amoxicillin).

Fluid accumulated in the middle ear for weeks can congeal into a chronic "glue ear" with hearing impairment, and repeated bouts of serous otitis in an adult, especially if unilateral, should raise the question of obstruction of the eustachian tube by tumor or lymphatic hypertrophy.

Split Earlobes

Presentation:

A patient will present with an earlobe split by a sudden pull on an earring or by prolonged traction from heavy earrings.

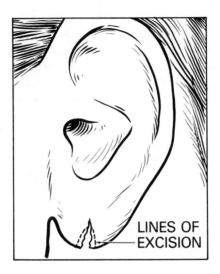

LINES OF EXCISION

What to do:

- Excise the skin edges on both sides of the wound, leaving the apical epithelium intact. Suture these freshened wound edges together using a fine monofilament material.
- Provide tetanus prophylaxis if needed (see p 277).

What not to do:

- Do not suture the wound primarily. The edges may epithelialize, resulting in the split redeveloping after the sutures are removed.

Discussion:

There are many techniques for the repair of split earlobes. Some methods, including this one, attempt to preserve the earring hole while others use a Z-plasty on the free margins of the lobes to prevent notching at the points of reunion. Depending on the specific circumstances, it may be advisable to consult with a plastic surgeon before attempting to repair this type of earlobe injury.

Epistaxis (Nose Bleed)

Presentation:

A patient generally arrives in the emergency department with active bleeding from his nose or spitting up blood that is draining into his throat. On occasion the hemorrhage has stopped but the patient is concerned because the bleeding has been recurring over the past few hours or days. Bleeding is most commonly visualized on the anterior aspect of the nasal septum within Kiesselbach's plexus. The anterior end of the inferior turbinate is another site where bleeding can be seen. Often, especially with posterior hemorrhaging, a specific bleeding site cannot be discerned.

What to do:

- Bring all equipment and supplies to the patient's bedside.
- Have the patient sit upright (unless hypotensive) and sedate the patient if necessary with a mild tranquilizer such as hydroxyzine (Vistaril). Cover the patient and yourself to protect your clothes.
- Prepare a solution of 5% cocaine or 2% tetracaine (Pontocaine) mixed 1:1 with 1% Neo-Synephrine or epinephrine 1:1000—a total of 5cc is usually sufficient.
- Form two elongated cotton pledgets and partially soak each in the solution.
- Have the patient blow the clots from his nose.
- Insert the medicated cotton pledgets as far back as possible into both nostrils.
- Have the patient relax with the pledgets in place for approximately 5–10 minutes. You may use this lull to ask about the patient's other medical problems.
- In the vast majority of cases, active bleeding will stop with this Tx alone, the cotton pledgets can be removed and the nasal cavity can be inspected using a nasal speculum and head lamp.
- If the bleeding point can be located, cauterize a 1cm area of mucosa around the bleeding site with a silver nitrate stick and then cauterize the site itself. Observe the patient for 15 minutes. If this stops the bleeding, cover the cauterized area with antibiotic ointment and instruct the patient in prevention (avoid picking the nose, bending over, sneezing, and straining) and treatment of recurrences (compress below the bridge of the nose with thumb and finger for five minutes).
- If the bleeding point cannot be located or if bleeding continues after cauterization, insert a Vaseline gauze anterior pack. To prevent putrification of the pack, cover the vaseline gauze with

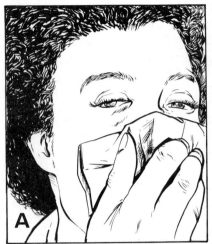
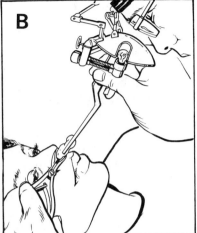

a tetracycline (Terramycin) ointment before insertion. Insert the gauze with bayonet forceps. Start with 3–4 plies layered accordian fashion on the floor of the nasal cavity, placing it as far posteriorly as possible, and pressing it down firmly with each subsequent layer. Continue inserting the gauze until the affected nasal cavity is tightly filled (expect to use about 3 to 5 feet of ½" gauze).

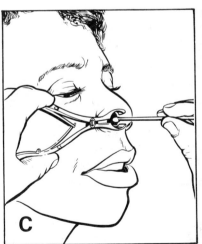
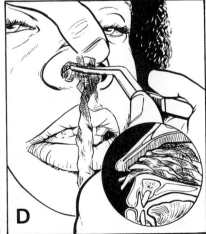

- Observe the patient for 15 minutes. If no further bleeding occurs (observe the posterior oropharynx), place the patient on a broad spectrum antibiotic (such as amoxicillin tid 250mg) for five days to help prevent a secondary sinusitis (cephalosporins are not well secreted in the mucus and thus are ineffective for prophylaxis here). The packing should be removed in 3 days.

- Instruct the patient against sneezing, bending over, straining, or nose picking. The patient's head should be kept elevated for 24–48 hours.
- If hemorrhage is suspected to have been severe, obtain orthostatic blood pressure and pulse recordings along with an hematocrit before making a disposition for the patient.
- If the hemorrhage does not stop after adequate packing anteriorly, then a simple posterior pack should be inserted, and the patient should be admitted to the hospital under the care of an otolaryngologist. A posterior bleeder can be tamponaded by inserting a Foley catheter (the catheter tip cut off) into the posterior nasopharynx and inflating the balloon with approximately 10cc of air or water. Place an anterior pack around the catheter in the usual manner, draw firm traction on the Foley catheter, tie a band of 1–0 silk at the point where the catheter protrudes through the packing, and then tie this string around a large gauze bolster so traction is maintained on the balloon.

What not to do:

- Do not waste time trying to locate a bleeding site while brisk bleeding obscures your vision in spite of vigorous suctioning. Have the patient blow out any clots and insert the medicated cotton pledgets.
- Do not get routine clotting studies unless there is other evidence of an underlying bleeding disorder.
- Do not cauterize or use instruments within the nose before providing adequate topical anesthesia (some initial blind suctioning may, however, be required to clear the nose of clots before instilling anesthetics).
- Do not discharge a patient as soon as the bleeding stops, but keep him in the ED for 15–30 minutes more. Posterior epistaxis typically stops and starts cyclically and may not be recognized until all the above treatments have failed.

Discussion:

Drying and crusting of the bleeding site, along with nose picking, may result in recurrent nasal hemorrhage. It may be helpful to instruct the patient on gently inserting Vaseline onto his nasal septum once or twice a day to prevent future drying and bleeding.

Nasal Foreign Bodies

Presentation:

Children may admit to parents that they have inserted something into their noses, but more often the history is obscure and the child presents with a purulent unilateral nasal discharge. Most commonly encountered are beans, beads, pebbles, paper wads, and eraser tips. These foreign bodies usually lodge on the floor of the anterior or middle third of the nasal cavity.

Occasionally, caustic material was sniffed into the nose or coughed up into the posterior nasopharynx (e.g., a ruptured tetracycline capsule), the patient will present with much discomfort and tearing, and inspection will reveal mucous membranes covered with particulate debris.

What to do:

- After initial inspection using a nasal speculum, suction out any purulent discharge and insert a cotton pledget soaked in a solution of one part phenylephrine (Neo-Synephrine) and one part tetracaine (Pontocaine) to shrink the nasal mucosa and provide local anesthesia. Remove the pledget after approximately 5 minutes.

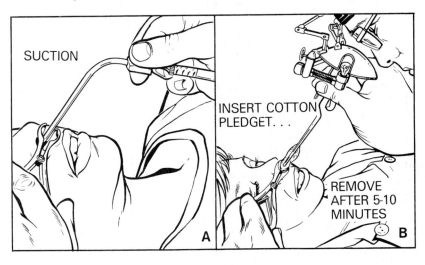

- If the patient is able to cooperate, have him try to blow his nose to remove the foreign body. With an infant it is sometimes possible to have the parent gently puff into the baby's mouth to blow the object out of the nose.

- Alligator forceps should be used to remove cloth, cotton, or paper foreign bodies. Pebbles, beans, and other hard foreign bodies are more easily grasped using bayonet forceps, or they may be rolled out using an ear curette, single skin hook, or right angle ear hook. An additional approach is to bypass the object with a fine Fogarty catheter, or small Foley catheter passing it superior to the FB, inflate the balloon and pull the object out through the nose.

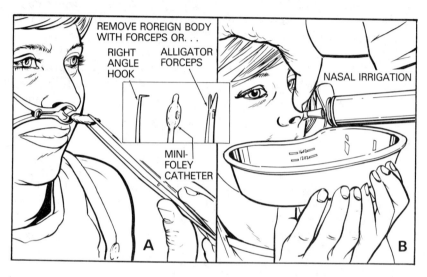

- To irrigate loose, light foreign bodies and particulate debris from the nasal cavity and posterior nasopharynx, simply insert

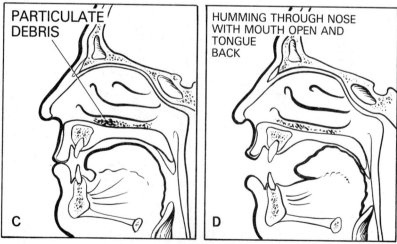

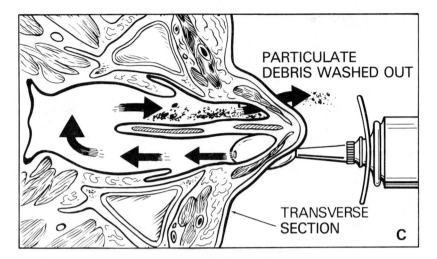

PARTICULATE
DEBRIS WASHED OUT

TRANSVERSE
SECTION   C

the bulbous nozzle of an irrigation syringe into one nostril, ask the patient to close off the back of his throat by repeating the sound "eng" and flush the irrigating solution out the opposite nostril.

- After the foreign body is removed, inspect the nasal cavity again and check for additional objects that may have been placed in the patient's nose.

What not to do:

- Do not ignore a unilateral nasal discharge in a child. It must be assumed to be secondary to a foreign body until proven otherwise.
- Do not push a foreign body down the back of a patient's throat, where it may be aspirated into the trachea.

Discussion:

The mucous membrane lining the nasal cavity allows you the tactical advantages of vasoconstriction and topical anesthesia. In cases where patients have unsuccessfully attempted to blow foreign bodies out of their noses, they may be successful after instillation of an anesthetic vasoconstriction solution. Cocaine is often preferred to Pontocaine as the topical anesthetic agent, but may be more difficult to keep in stock.

Nasal Fractures

Presentation:

After a direct blow to the nose the patient usually arives at the emergency department with minimal continued hemorrhage. There is usually tender ecchymotic swelling over the nasal bones or the anterior maxillary spine; inspection and palpation may (or not) disclose nasal deformity.

What to do:

- Instill cotton pledgets soaked in 5% cocaine or 2% tetracaine (Pontocaine) mixed 1:1 with 1% Neo-Synephrine or epinephrine 1:1000 into both nasal cavities.
- Examine for any associated injuries (i.e., blowout fractures).
- Send the patient for x rays of the nasal bones.
- After removing the cotton pledgets, inspect the nasal mucosa for large lacerations or a septal hematoma.
- Patients with nondisplaced fractures without deformity should be sent home with analgesics, cold packs, and instructions to avoid contact sports and related activities for six weeks.
- Patients with displaced fractures and/or nasal deformity should have otolaryngologic or plastic surgery consultation for immediate or delayed reduction. Patients can be instructed that reduction is more accurate after the swelling subsides and there is no greater difficulty if it is done within six days of the injury.
- Septal hematomas should be drained to prevent septal necrosis and the development of a saddle nose deformity. Otolaryngologic consultation is advisable.
- There is only the need to reassure the patient with an isolated fracture of the anterior nasal spine (in the columella), without restricting their activities.
- A laceration over a nasal fracture should probably be closed with antibiotic prophylaxis (e.g., penicillin VK 500mg po qid for 5 days).

What not to do:

- Do not assume a negative x ray means no fracture when a deformity is apparent. X rays can often be inaccurate in determining the presence and nature of a nasal fracture. Always rely on your clinical judgement if a fracture is suspected.
- Do not pack an injured nose that does not continue to bleed significantly. Packing is generally unnecessary and will only add to the patient's discomfort.

Sinusitis

Presentation:

The patient will usually complain of a dull pain in the face, gradually increasing over a couple of days, exacerbated by any jerky motion of the head, and perhaps radiating to the upper molar teeth (via the maxillary antrum), or eye (via ethmoid). Often there is a sensation of facial congestion and stuffiness.

Many patients (and physicians) have been conditioned by the advertising of over-the-counter antihistamines for "sinus" problems (usually meaning "allergic rhinitis"), and may relate a long history of "sinusitis" which, on closer questioning, turns out to have been no such thing.

Transillumination of sinuses in the ED is often unrewarding, but you may elicit tenderness over the maxillary or frontal sinuses or between the eyes (ethmoid sinuses). Swelling and erythema may exist and you may even see pus draining below the nasal turbinates. The patient's voice may have a resonance similar to that of a "stopped up" nose.

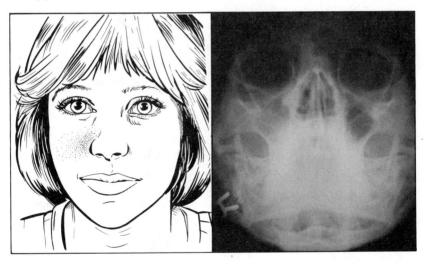

What to do:

- Rule out other causes of facial pain or headache via history (did the patient wake up with a migraine or develop eyestrain in the evening?) and physical examination (palpate scalp muscles, temporal arteries, temperomandibular joints, eyes, and teeth).
- Demonstration of acute sinusitis often requires x rays, but you can usually get adequate visualization of maxillary, frontal,

and ethmoid sinuses with one upright Water's view. Chronic sinusitis appears as thickened mucosa; acute as an air-fluid level.

- Shrink swollen nasal mucosa (and thereby open the ostia draining the sinuses) with 1% phenylephrine (Neo-Synephrine) nose drops. Drip 2 drops in each nostril, have the patient lie supine 2 minutes, and then repeat the process (this allows the first application to open the anterior nose so the second gets farther back). Have the patient repeat this process every 4 hours, but for no more than three days (to avoid rhinitis medicamentosum).

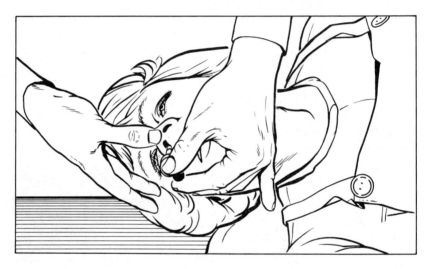

- Add systemic sympathomimetic decongestants (e.g., pseudephedrine 60mg q6h).
- If there is fever, pus, heat, or any other sign of a bacterial superinfection, add antibiotics (e.g., penicillin VK 500mg q6h or amoxicillin 500mg q8h x 10 days).
- Arrange for followup.

What not to do:

- Do not prescribe antihistamines, which can make mucous secretions dry and thick, and interfere with necessary drainage. Antihistamines only cure sinusitis on television, or when it is due to allergic rhinitis.
- Do not allow patients to use decongestant nose drops more than 3 days, thereby allowing their nasal mucosa to become habituated to sympathomimetic medication. When they stop the drops they will suffer a rebound nasal congestion (rhinitis med-

icamentosum) which requires time, topical steroids, and reeducation to resolve.

- Do not prescribe topical or systemic sympathomimetic decongestants to a patient who suffers from hypertension, tachycardia, jitters, or difficulty initiating urination, all of which may be exacerbated.

Discussion:

The paranasal sinuses drain through tiny ostia under the nasal turbinates which, if occluded, allow secretions and pressure to build up, resulting in pressure and pain of acute sinusitis, and the air-fluid levels visible on upright x rays. Bacterial superinfection can spread from the ethmoid sinuses into periorbital tissue, and from frontal and sphenoid sinuses into the CSF and venous cavernous sinus. If the treatment above does not reestablish normal sinus drainage via the ostia, surgical drainage may be required during followup.

Rarely, you may encounter an acute amebic sinusitis, usually frontal, and caused by *Naegleria* acquired by swimming in contaminated, warm, fresh water. This differs from common or garden variety bacterial sinusitis by its sudden onset over a few hours, and its rapid progression over hours or days to fatal meningioencephalitis.

Pharyngitis (Sore Throat)

Presentation:

The patient complains of pain in the throat, exacerbated by swallowing. (It is important to differentiate pain on swallowing (odynophagia) from difficulty swallowing (dysphagia), the latter being more likely caused by obstruction or abnormal muscular movement.) There may or may not be symptoms of an upper respiratory infection.

There may be diffuse redness of the oral pharynx, enlarged tonsils or other lymphoid tissue, or lymphoid hyperplasia "cobblestoning" of the posterior pharyngeal wall. Tonsillar crypts may be enlarged and purulent, making spots of yellow pus over the tonsils, or the tonsils may be covered with a dirty-looking exudate.

Pharyngitis which is worse upon rising in the morning, coupled with a runny nose, hoarse voice, and cough, suggests a primary problem of rhinitis, with mucus drainage producing the other symptoms. Pharyngitis associated with conjunctivitis, adenopathy, myalgias, rash, and malaise suggests a viral etiology.

What to do:

- First examine the ears, nose, and mouth, which are, after all, connected to the pharynx, and often contain clues to the diagnosis.
- Depress the tongue with a blade, have the patient raise his soft palate by saying "ah," inspect the posterior pharynx, and swab both tonsillar pillars for a culture. (You can decide later whether you really need to plant the culture.)
- If you are in the middle of an epidemic of group A streptococcal pharyngitis; if the patient is between 3 and 25 years old, has a history of rheumatic fever and recurrent "strep throats" and has been exposed; and if the patient has a red throat, fever, tender anterior cervical nodes, and no viral URI symptoms (or any convincing subset of the above); give him 1,200,000 units of benzathene penicillin im, and do not bother planting the culture. The next best treatment (for the shot-shy) is oral penicillin, VK 250mg q6h for 10 days, or erythromycin for the penicillin-allergic. (Use ½ dose for children 5–10 yrs.)
- If culture results will be back in a day, the patient can be contacted, and you are willing to take responsibility for the followup, or if you doubt a group A streptococcus infection, you may prefer to postpone antibiotic eradication of any group A streptococcus until the throat culture demonstrates the infection.

  There are no reliable clinical markers of group A streptococcal infection. Typically, only about a quarter of cultures will return positive, and half of those positives are only carriers, who do not raise their anti-strep titers after the episode of pharyngitis.
- If the patient has performed fellatio in the previous week or two, you should also plate the throat swab on Thayer-Martin agar. Doses of penicillin used to eradicate streptococcus are usually not high enough to cure gonococcal pharyngitis (use 4.8 million units of procaine penicillin im and 1gm of probenecid po).
- If you suspect mononucleosis, draw blood for atypical lymphocytes and a heterophile or monospot to confirm the diagnosis.
- Relieve pain with aspirin, warm saline gargles, and gargles or lozenges containing phenol as a mucosal anesthetic (e.g., Chloraseptic, Cepastat). Viscous Xylocaine gargles are a last resort.

What not to do:

- Do not miss an acute epiglottitis or supraglottitis. In a child, this presents as a sudden, severe pharyngitis, with a gutteral, rather than hoarse voice (because it hurts to speak), drooling (because it hurts to swallow), and respiratory distress (because swelling narrows the airway). Adults usually have a more gradual onset, over several days, and are not as prone to a sudden airway occlusion, unless they present later in the progression of the swelling, already with some respiratory distress.
- Do not give ampicillin to a patient with mononucleosis. The resulting rash helps make the diagnosis, and does not imply ampicillin allergy, but can be uncomfortable.
- Do not miss abscesses, which usually require hospitalization and intravenous penicillin, if not drainage. Peritonsillar abcesses or cellulitis make the tonsillar pillar bulge towards the midline. Retropharyngeal abscesses (and epiglottitis) may require soft tissue lateral neck films to visualize.
- Do not miss the rare but deadly causes of sore throat. A patient with paresthesia at the site of an old, healed bite and painful spasms when he even thinks of swallowing may have rabies. A patient with facial palsy, myocarditis, and a tough, white, membrane adherent to the posterior pharynx may have diptheria. You cannot diagnose them unless you think of them.

Discussion:

The general public knows to see a doctor for a sore throat, but the actual benefit of this visit is unclear. Rheumatic fever is a sequela of about 1% of group A streptococcal infections, and only about 10% of sore throats seen by physicians represent group A streptococcal infections. Post-streptococcal glomerulonephritis is usually a self-limiting illness. It is far from clear that penicillin therapy does anything to reduce symptoms or shorten the course of a sore throat, but it probably does inhibit progress of the infection into tonsillitis, peritonsillar and retropharyngeal abscesses, adenitis, and pneumonia.

Foreign Body in Throat

Presentation:

The patient thinks he recently swallowed a fish or a chicken bone, pop top from an old-style can, or something of the sort, and still can feel a foreign body sensation in his throat, especially (perhaps painfully) when swallowing. The patient may be able to localize the FB sensation precisely above the thyroid cartilage (implying an FB in the hypopharynx you may be able to see), or he may only vaguely localize the FB sensation to the suprasternal notch (which could imply an FB anywhere in the esophagus). An FB in the tracheobronchial tree usually stimulates coughing and wheezing. Obstruction of the esophagus produces drooling and spitting up of whatever is swallowed.

What to do:

- Establish exactly what was swallowed, when, and the progression of symptoms since then.
- Test the patient's ability to swallow, using a small cup of water and small piece of bread. See what symptoms are reproduced, and watch for aspiration.
- Percuss and auscultate the patient's chest. An FB sensation in the throat can be produced by a pneumothorax, pneumomediastinum, or esophageal disease, all of which may show up on a chest x ray.
- Inspect the oropharynx with a tongue depressor, looking for FBs or abrasions.
- Inspect the hypopharynx with a headlamp and mirror, paying special attention to the base of the tongue and vallecula, where FBs are likely to lodge. Maximize your visibility and minimize gagging by holding the patient's tongue out (use a washcloth or 4" × 4" gauze for traction and take care not to lacerate the frenulum of the tongue on the lower incisors) and have the patient raise his soft palate by panting "like a dog." This may be accomplished without topical anesthesia, but if the patient is skeptical or tends to gag, you may anesthetize the soft palate and posterior pharynx with a spray (e.g., Cetacaine or 10% lidocaine) or by having the patient gargle with viscous Xylocaine diluted 1:1 with tap water. Some patients may continue to gag with the entire pharynx anesthetized.
- If you find an FB to pluck out (with bayonet forceps) or an abrasion of the mucosa, you may have diagnosed the problem. Further treatment is probably not required, but you should instruct the patient to seek followup if pain worsens, fever

develops, breathing or swallowing is difficult, or if the FB sensation has not totally resolved in 2 days.

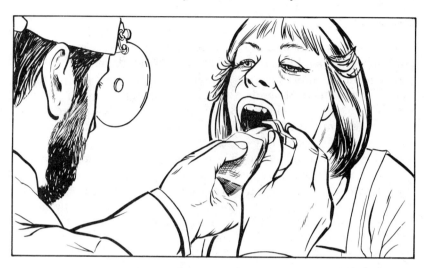

- If you and your patient are not satisfied, you may proceed to a soft tissue lateral x ray of the neck. This will probably not show radiolucent or small FBs, such as fish bones, or aluminum pop tops, but may point out other pathology, such as a retropharyngeal abscess, Zenker's diverticulum, or severe cervical spondylosis, which might account for symptoms (and also allows some time for the patient's gag reflex to settle down, in case you were not able to inspect the hypopharynx on the first try).
- You may also want to proceed to a barium swallow, if available, to demonstrate with fluoroscopy any problems with swallowing motility, or perhaps coat and thus visualize a radiolucent FB. A barium swallow is definitely indicated if the patient has signs of esophageal obstruction.
- Reserve laryngoscopy, esophagoscopy, and bronchoscopy under general anesthesia for the few cases where your suspicion of a perforating FB remains high.

What not to do:

- Do not reassure the patient that you have ruled out an FB if you have not. Instead, explain that undetected FBs (or the symptoms of an undetected abrasion) are likely to resolve spontaneously, and that further workup involves unwarranted risk, discomfort, and expense.

- Do not miss preexisting pathology incidentally discovered during swallowing.

Discussion:

The narrowest strait in most gastrointestinal tracts, and thus the spot where most FBs hang up after passing through the hypopharynx, is in the proximal esophagus. This narrowing is posterior to the thyroid cartilage and under the constrictor pharyngis inferior (or cricopharyngeal) muscle. Unfortunately, there is no safe, easy way to see into the proximal esophagus (usually, a long, rigid esophagoscope is used). It is thus almost impossible to rule out a small FB perforating the esophagus which could, (but seldom does), develop into a disastrous mediastinitis. Routine triple endoscopy, under general anesthesia, poses a greater risk than watchful waiting for the great majority of patients who safely pass esophageal FBs or whose symptoms were due to an abrasion.

The sensation of a lump in the throat, unrelated to swallowing food or drink, may be globus hystericus, which is related to cricopharyngeal spasm and anxiety. The initial workup is the same as with any FB sensation in the throat.

A pill, composed of irritating medicine, and swallowed without adequate liquid, may hang up in the throat and cause ulceration of the mucosa of the pharynx or esophagus. Bay leaves, invisible on x rays and laryngoscopy, have lodged in the esophagus at the cricopharyngeus and produced severe symptoms until removed via rigid esophagoscopy.

Mononucleosis (Glandular Fever)

Presentation:

The patient is usually of school age (nursery through night school) and complains of several days of fever, malaise, lassitude, myalgias, and anorexia, culminating in a severe sore throat.

The physical examination is remarkable for generalized lymphadenopathy, including the anterior and posterior cervical chains and huge tonsils, perhaps meeting in the midline and covered with a dirty-looking exudate. There may also be palatal petechiae and swelling, splenomegaly, hepatomegaly, and a diffuse maculopapular rash.

What to do:

- Perform a complete physical examination, looking for signs of other ailments, and the rare complication of airway obstruction, encephalitis, hemolytic anemia, thrombocytopenic purpura, myocarditis, pericarditis, hepatitis, and rupture of the spleen.
- Send off blood tests, either a differential white cell count (looking for atypical lymphocytes) or a heterophil or mono spot test. Either of these tests, along with the generalized lymphadenopathy, confirms the diagnosis of mononucleosis, but atypical lymphocytes are more likely to be present acutely.
- Culture the throat. Patients with mononucleosis harbor group A streptococcus and require penicillin with about the same frequency as anyone else with a sore throat.
- Warn the patient that the convalescence is longer than that of most viral illnesses (typically 2–4 weeks, occasionally more), and that he should seek attention in case of lightheadedness, abdominal or shoulder pain, or any other sign of the rare complications above.
- Arrange for medical followup.

What not to do:

- Do not routinely give penicillin for the pharyngitis, and certainly do not give ampicillin. In a patient with mononucleosis, ampicillin can produce an uncomfortable rash, which, incidentally, does not imply allergy to ampicillin.
- Do not unnecessarily frighten the patient about splenic rupture. If the spleen is clinically enlarged, he should avoid contact sports, but spontaneous ruptures are rare.
- Do not agonize over locating the source. With an incubation period of one to two months, it is usually impossible to find the (usually oral) contact.

Discussion:

All of the above probably apply to cytomegalovirus as well, although the severe tonsillitis and positive heterophil test are both less likely. Some who report having mono twice probably actually had CMV once and mono once.

4

Oral/Dental

Temporomandibular Joint Arthritis

Presentation:

The patient usually complains of pain and popping or crackling sounds in the ear when chewing, or may complain of the less obvious symptoms of pain in the side of the face or down the carotid sheath, tinnitus, dizziness, decreased hearing, itching, or a foreign body sensation in the external ear canal.

There is usually tenderness to palpation over the temporomandibular joint but another common presentation is that of a recurrent external otitis: low intensity pain the the temporomandibular joint is felt as itching in the external ear canal, prompting the patient to scratch with a swab, abrading the epithelium, and allowing bacteria to invade.

Patients may have been previously diagnosed as suffering from migraines or sinusitis.

Predisposing factors include malocclusion, recent extensive dental work, or a habit of grinding the teeth (bruxism), all of which put unusual stress upon the TM joint.

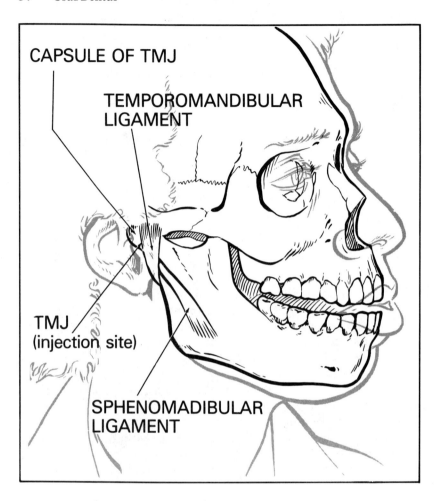

CAPSULE OF TMJ

TEMPOROMANDIBULAR LIGAMENT

TMJ
(injection site)

SPHENOMADIBULAR LIGAMENT

What to do:

- Examine the head thoroughly for other causes of the pain, including visual acuity, cranial nerves, and palpation of the scalp muscles and the temporal arteries. Pain and popping on moving the TMJ is a useful but not infallible sign. Look for signs of bruxism, such as ground-down teeth.
- If pain is severe, you may try injecting the TMJ, just anterior to the tragus, with 1ml of plain lidocaine. If this helps, you may have made the diagnosis, but done little for long-term relief.
- Explain to the patient the pathophysiology of the syndrome: how many different symptoms may be produced by inflammation at one joint, how TMJ arthritis is not necessarily related to arthritis at other joints, how common it is (some estimates are as high as 20% of the population).

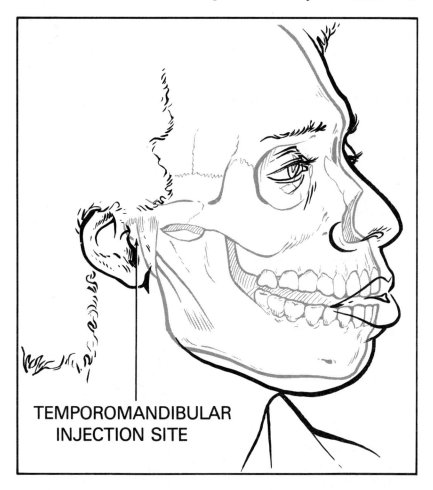

TEMPOROMANDIBULAR
INJECTION SITE

- Prescribe anti-inflammatory analgesics (e.g., aspirin, Motrin), a soft diet, heat, and muscle relaxants (e.g., Valium) if necessary for muscle spasm.
- Refer the patient for followup to a dentist or otolaryngologist who has some interest in and experience with TMJ arthritis. Long-term treatments include bite blocks to prevent malocclusion and bruxism, orthodontic correction, biofeedback, and elimination of other precipitating factors.

What not to do:

- Do not rule out TMJ arthritis simply because the joint is not tender on your examination. This syndrome typically fluctuates, and the diagnosis often is made on history alone.
- Do not omit the TMJ in your workup of any headache.

Discussion:

Perhaps everyone suffers pain in the TMJ occasionally, and only a few require treatment or modification of lifestyle to reduce symptoms. In the ED the diagnosis of TMJ arthritis is often suspected, but seldom made definitively. It can be gratifying, however, to see patients with myriads of seemingly unrelated symptoms, or other diagnoses altogether, respond dramatically after only conservative measures and advice.

Jaw Dislocation

Presentation:

The patient's jaw is "out" and will not close, usually following a yawn, less often following trauma or a dystonic reaction.

What to do:

- If there was no trauma (and especially if the patient is a chronic dislocator) proceed directly to attempt reduction. If there is any possibility of an associated fracture, obtain x rays first.
- Have the patient sit on a low stool, his back and head braced against something firm—either against the wall, facing you, or in front of you, the back of his head braced against your legs.
- Wrap your thumbs in gauze, seat them upon the lower molars, grasp both sides of the mandible, lock your elbows, and, bending from the waist, exert slow, steady pressure down and back.
- If the jaw does not relocate convincingly, you may want to reassess the dislocation with x rays, and try again using intravenous diazepam to overcome the muscle spasm and intraarticular lidocaine to overcome the pain. (See p 84.)
- After reducing the dislocation it will be comforting to apply a soft cervical collar to reduce the range of motion at the TMJ.

What not to do:

- Try not to get your thumbs bitten when the jaw snaps back.
- Do not put pressure on oral prostheses that could cause them to break.

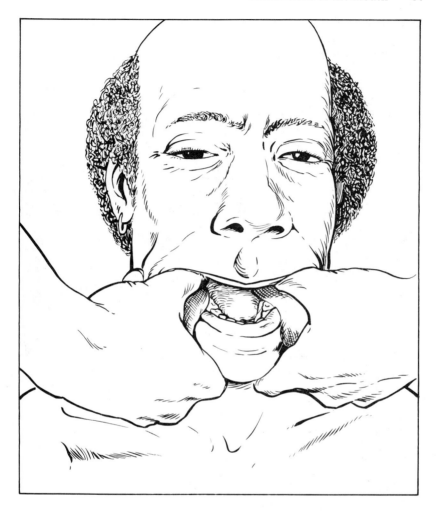

Discussion:

The mandible can only dislocate anteriorly, but does so every time the jaw is opened wide. Dislocation is often a chronic problem (avoided by limiting motion) and associated with temporomandibular joint arthritis (see p 83).

Lacerations of the Mouth

Presentation:

Because of the rich vascularity of the soft tissues of the mouth, impact injuries often lead to dramatic hemorrhages that send patients to the emergency department with relatively trivial lacerations. Blunt trauma to the face can cause secondary lacerations of the lips, frenulum, buccal mucosa, gingiva, and tongue. Active bleeding has almost always stopped by the time a patient with a minor laceration has reached the emergency department.

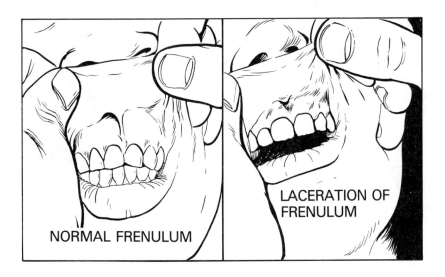

NORMAL FRENULUM

LACERATION OF FRENULUM

What to do:

- Provide appropriate tetanus prophylaxis and check for associated injuries such as loose teeth, mandibular or facial fractures.
- When only small lacerations are present and only minimal gaping of the wound occurs, reassurance and simple aftercare is all that is required. Let the patient or parents know that you realize how frightening all that blood looks when it is coming out of the mouth. Minimize any embarrassment the patient might have regarding the hospital visit. Let him know the wound will become somewhat uncomfortable and covered with pus over the next 48 hours and tell him to rinse with water or half strength hydrogen peroxide after meals and every one to two hours.
- If the wound edges gape significantly or there is a flap or deformity when the underlying musculature contracts, the wound should first be anesthetized and loosely approximated using a 4–0 or 5–0 absorbable suture. A traction stitch or special rubber-tipped clamp can be very helpful when attempting to suture the tongue of a small child or intoxicated adult. The same aftercare as above applies.

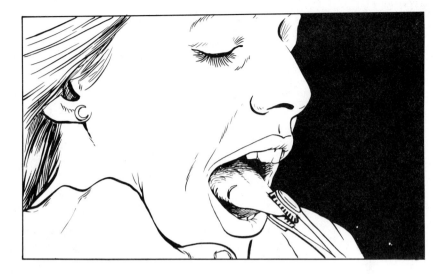

- When the exterior surface of the lip is lacerated, any separation of the underlying musculature must be repaired with buried absorbable sutures. To avoid an unsightly scar when the lip heals, precise skin approximation is very important. One must first approximate the vermilion border, making this the key suture. Fine non-absorbable suture material (e.g., 6–0 nylon or Prolene) is most appropriate for the skin surfaces of the lip while a fine absorbable suture (e.g., 6–0 Dexon or Vicryl) is quite acceptable on the mucosa and vermilion.
- When deep lacerations of the mucosa or lacerations of the lip occur, prophylactic penicillin (500mg penicillin VK qid x 3–4 days) is considered appropriate for preventing deep tissue infections. Penicillin prophylaxis should be provided for any sutured mouth laceration.

What not to do:

- Do not bother to repair a simple laceration/avulsion of the frenulum of the upper lip. This will heal quite nicely on its own.
- Do not use non-absorbable suture material on the tongue, gingiva or buccal mucosa. There is no advantage and suture removal on a small child will be an unpleasant struggle at best.

Discussion:

Imprecise repair of the vermilion border will lead to a "step-off" or puckering that is unsightly and difficult to repair later on.

Aphthous Ulcer (Canker Sore)

Presentation:

The patient will complain of a very painful lesion in the mouth, and may be worried about having herpes. A pale yellow, flat, even-bordered ulcer on an erythematous base may be seen on the buccal or labial mucosa, lingual sulci, soft palate, pharynx, tongue, or gingiva. Lesions are usually solitary, but can be multiple and recurrent.

What to do:

- Attempt to differentiate from lesions of herpes simplex (see below) and reassure the patient of the benign nature of most canker sores.
- Inform the patient that these lesions usually last 1–2 weeks.
- For pain relief, try tetracycline elixir (or tablets dissolved in water) not swallowed, but applied to lesions or used as a mouth wash (why this works is unclear). Benadryl elixir, Xylocaine 2% Viscous Solution, and Orabase HCA applied topically, also can provide symptomatic relief.

Discussion:

These lesions have no known etiology, but can be precipitated by trauma, food allergy, stress, and systemic illness. Recurrent aphthous ulcers may accompany malignancy or autoimmune disease. At present, the treatment is only palliative, and may not alter the course of the syndrome.

Herpangina and hand-foot-and-mouth disease can produce lesions indistinguishable from aphthous ulcers, but which are instead part of coxsackie viral exanthems, usually occurring in clusters among children.

Oral Herpes Simplex (Cold Sore)

Presentation:

The patient will have burning or soreness at an intra- or extraoral lesion consisting of clusters of small vesicles on an erythematous base, which then rupture to produce red ulcerations with crusting or superinfection. These lesions occur intraorally on the hard palate or gingiva or, more commonly, extraorally at the vermilion border of the lip.

What to do:

- Scrape the base of a vesicle (warn the patient this hurts) smear on a slide, stain with Wright's or Giemsa, and examine for multinucleate giant cells (look for nuclear molding). This is called a Tzanck Prep, and establishes the diagnosis of herpes.

- Topical acyclovir (Zovirax) reduces viral shedding, but has not been shown to benefit oral herpes simplex. (Oral or intravenous preparations may be more efficacious.)

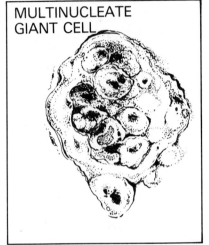

MULTINUCLEATE GIANT CELL

- Topical Orabase, or Xylocaine 2% Viscous Solution may relieve the pain.
- Instruct the patient to keep lesions clean, and avoid touching lesions (so as not to spread the virus to eyes, unaffected skin, and other people).
- Inform the patient that oral herpes need not be related to genital herpes; that the vesicles and pain should resolve over about two weeks (barring superinfection); that they are infectious during this period (and perhaps other times as well); and that the herpes simplex virus, residing in sensory ganglia, can be expected to cause recurrences from time to time (especially during illness or stress).

Discussion:

Home remedies for cold sores include ether, lecithin, lysine, and vitamin E. Because herpes is a self-limiting affliction, all work, but, in controlled studies, none have outperformed placebos (which also do very well).

Sialolithiasis (Salivary Duct Stones)

Presentation:

Patients of any age may develop salivary duct stones. The vast

majority of such stones occur in Wharton's duct from the submax-
illary gland. The patient will be alarmed by the rapid swelling
beneath his jaw that suddenly appears while he is eating. The
swelling may be painful but is not hot or erythematous and usually
subsides within 2 hours. This swelling may only be intermittent and
may not occur with every meal.

Infection can occur and will be accompanied by increased pain,
exquisite tenderness, erythema and fever. Under these circumstances pus can sometimes be expressed from the opening of the
duct when the gland is pressed open.

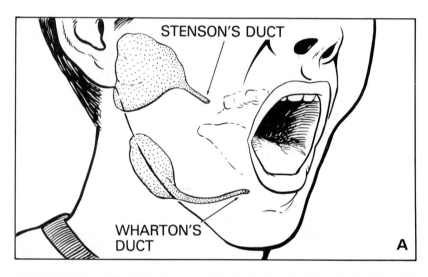

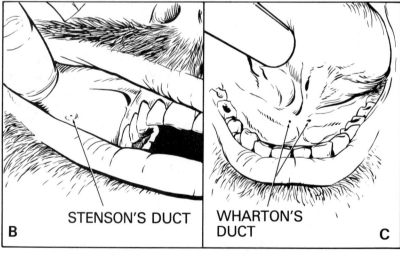

What to do:

- Bimanually palpate the course of the salivary duct, feeling for stones.
- When a small superficial stone can be felt, anesthetize the tissue beneath the duct and ampule with a small amount of lidocaine 1% with epinephrine. If available, a punctum dilator can be used to widen the orifice of the duct. Then milk the gland and duct with your fingers to express the stone(s).
- If the stone cannot be palpated, try to locate it with x rays. Standard x rays of the mandible are likely to demonstrate only large stones. Dental x ray film shot at right angles to the floor of the mouth is much more likely to demonstrate small stones in Wharton's duct. Place film between cheek and gum to visualize Stenson's duct.
- When a stone cannot be demonstrated or cannot be manually expressed, the patient should be referred for contrast sialography and/or surgical removal of the stone. Often sialography will show whether an obstruction is due to stenosis, a stone, or a tumor.
- Begin treatment of any infection with Dicloxacillin 500mg po qid x 10 days after obtaining cultures.

What not to do:

- Do not attempt to dilate a salivary duct if mumps is suspected. Acute, *persistent* pain and swelling of the parotid gland along with inflammation of the papilla of Stenson's duct, fever, lymphocytosis hyperamylasemia and malaise should alert the examiner to the probability of mumps.

Discussion:

Salivary duct stones are generally composed of calcium carbonate and calcium phosphate. Although the majority form in Wharton's duct in the floor of the mouth, approximately 10% occur in Stenson's duct in the cheek, and 5% in the sublingual ducts. Depending on the location and the size of the stone the presenting symptoms will vary. As a rule though, the onset of swelling will be sudden and associated with salivation during a meal.

Dental Trauma

Presentation:

After a direct blow to the mouth the patient may have a portion of a tooth broken off, a tooth may be loosened to a variable degree, or there may be a complete avulsion of a tooth from its socket.

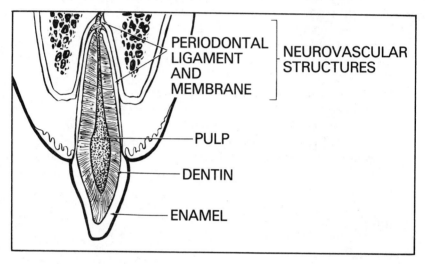

What to do:

- Prehospital care should include storing the tooth under the patient's tongue or between the gums and cheek.
- Assess the patient for any associated injuries such as facial or mandibular fractures.
- For chipped or fractured teeth, cover the exposed surface with tooth varnish (copal ether varnish) or clear nail polish to decrease sensitivity. Instruct the patient to avoid hot and cold food or drink and inform him that the tooth may die from even small fractures and require root canal therapy at a later date.
- When fractures are through the pulp chamber or close to it, get an early dental consultation.
- Very loose teeth should be wired for stability, and the patient should be informed that root canal work may be necessary. Dental consultation is often required for tooth stabilization.
- An avulsed tooth should be gently rinsed with normal saline and the socket irrigated, then the tooth should be grasped between thumb and index finger with a dry 2" × 2" gauze sponge and immediately reinserted by pressing firmly but

slowly until the tooth is fixed in place. A partially extracted tooth can be pushed into place without first irrigating the tooth and socket. The tooth should then be fixed into place with a temporary figure 8 suture over the tooth or with wiring to an adjacent stable tooth. The patient should be advised to seek early dental followup as root canal therapy will be required if the tooth stays in place.

What not to do:

- Do not clean or debride small fragments of periodontal fibers attached to the root of an avulsed tooth.
- Do not delay inserting an avulsed tooth into its socket for any reason.
- Do not replant avulsed primary deciduous teeth. They are too difficult to stabilize.

Discussion:

The most significant factor in determining the success or failure of a replaced tooth is the length of time elapsed prior to replantation. The chance for success is dramatically reduced 30 minutes after avulsion. Reimplanted teeth may survive for many years, but usually not as long as their uninjured neighbors, and may require root canal therapy soon after replacement. The aim of early replacement is not to preserve the pulp, but to preserve the periodontal membrane and ligament.

Bleeding After Dental Surgery

Presentation:

The patient had an extraction or other dental surgery performed earlier in the day, now has bleeding at the site, and cannot reach his dentist.

What to do:

- Ask what procedure was done.
- Using suction and saline irrigation, clear any packing and clot from the bleeding site.
- Roll a 2″ × 2″ gauze pad, insert it over the bleeding site, and

have the patient apply constant pressure upon it (biting down usually suffices) for 10 minutes.
- If this does not stop the bleeding, pack the bleeding site with Gelfoam, with gauze soaked in topical thrombin, or with bone wax (if the site is a bony socket), place the gauze pad on top, and apply pressure again.
- An arterial bleeder resistant to all the above may require ligation with a figure eight stitch.
- Assess any possible large blood loss with orthostatic vital signs.
- When the bleeding stops, remove the overlying gauze, have the patient leave the site alone for a day, and see his dentist in followup.

What not to do:

- Do not routinely obtain laboratory clotting studies or hematocrits, unless there is a suspicion that they should be abnormal.

Discussion:

Occasionally, this problem can be handled over the telephone. Some say a tea bag works even better than a gauze pad.

Dental Pain Post Extraction (Dry Socket)

Presentation:

The patient develops severe pain two to three days following an extraction. The pain is often excruciating and is not relieved by oral analgesics. There may be an associated foul odor and taste.

What to do:

- Irrigate the socket with normal saline.
- Pack the socket with ¼" gauze soaked in oil of cloves (eugenol).
- Prescribe a codeine or oxycodone (hydrochloride) analgesic for additional pain relief.
- Refer the patient back to his dentist for followup.

Discussion:

Dry socket results from a pathologic process combining loss of the healing blood clot with a localized inflammation or infection (osteitis or osteomyelitis).

Dental Pain—Pulpitis

Presentation:

The patient develops an acute toothache with sharp and throbbing pain. The patient may or may not be aware of having a cavity in that tooth. Initially the pain is decreased by heat and increased by cold, but as the condition progresses, heat makes the pain worse, while ice will dramatically relieve it. Physical exam may reveal a dental cavity (caries) without facial or gingival swelling.

What to do:

- Administer a strong analgesic such as oxycodone in combination with acetaminophen or aspirin (Percocet, Percodan) and prescribe additional medication for home use.
- If a cavity is present, insert a small cotton pledget soaked in oil of cloves (eugenol). The cotton should fill the cavity without rising above the opening (where it would strike the opposing tooth).
- Refer the patient to a dentist within 12 hours for definitive therapy (removal of caries, removal of pulp, or removal of the tooth).

What not to do:

- Do not occlude the caries with cotton if there is any purulent drainage or facial swelling.

Discussion:

As a patient's condition progresses from pulpitis to pulpal necrosis, the patient experiences excruciating pain caused by fluid and gaseous pressure within a closed space. Heat increases the volume and hence the pain, while cold reduces it.

Dental Pain—Abscess

Presentation:

The patient complains of facial/dental pain with facial swelling and cellulitis associated with varying degrees of systemic toxicity. Percussion of the offending tooth will elicit increased pain, while dental caries may or may not be apparent. There may be a fluctuant abscess detected by an examining finger in the soft tissues of the mouth, face, or neck.

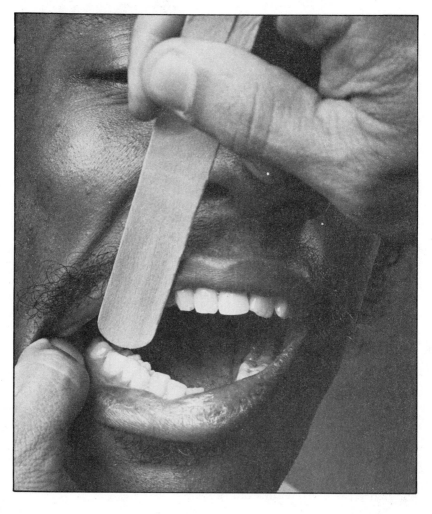

What to do:

- Adequate pain medication should be administered and prescribed for continued pain relief. A combination of aspirin or acetaminophen with codeine or oxycodone usually suffices.
- Depending on the level of toxicity, the patient should initially either be treated with parenteral or oral penicillin, and a 10-day course should be prescribed.
- If a fluctuant abscess cavity is present, then incision and drainage at the most dependent location is necessary and, when possible, a drain should be inserted for 24 hours.
- Patients should be instructed to apply warm compresses to the affected area and seek followup care from a dentist within 24 hours.

What not to do:

- Do not insert an obstructing pack (i.e. cotton soaked with oil of cloves) into a tooth cavity when an abscess or cellulitis is present.

Discussion:

More serious complications and infections, such as Ludwig's angina, cavernous sinus thrombosis, and osteomyelitis, must always be kept in mind.

Dental Pain—Pericoronitis

Presentation:

The patient is aged 17–25 and seeks help because of painful swelling and infection around an erupting or impacted third molar (wisdom tooth). Occasionally, there can be trismus or pain on biting. The site appears red and swollen with a flap that may reveal a partial tooth eruption and purulent drainage when pulled open.

What to do:

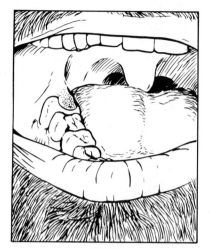

- Irrigate with a weak (2%) hydrogen peroxide solution. Purulent material can be released by placing the catheter tip of the irrigating syringe under the tissue flap overlying the impacted molar.
- Prescribe oral analgesics for comfort as well as penicillin over the next 10 days penicillin VK 250–500mg qid).
- Instruct the patient on the importance of cleansing away any food particles that collect beneath the gingival flap. This can be accomplished by simply using a soft toothbrush or by using water jet irrigation.
- A dental followup should be provided to observe the resolution of the acute infection and to evaluate the need for removal of the molar.

Gingivitis

Presentation:

The patient will complain of generalized severe pain, often with a foul taste or odor. The gingiva will appear edematous and red with a grayish necrotic membrane between the teeth.

What to do:

- Prescribe penicillin VK (250mg qid) for ten days.
- Instruct the patient to use warm saline rinses, every one to two hours along with gentle brushing using sodium bicarbonate powder.
- For comfort, prescribe viscous lidocaine.
- For definitive care and the prevention of periodontal disease refer the patient for dental followup care.

Oral Candidiasis (Thrush)

Presentation:

An infant (usually with a concurrent diaper rash) will have white patches in his mouth, or an older patient (usually with poor oral hygiene, diabetes, or some immunodeficiency) will complain of a sore mouth. On physical examination, there is intense, red inflammation throughout the oral cavity, and probably some white patches which wipe off easily with a swab.

What to do:

- Confirm the diagnosis by smearing the exudate, Gram staining, and examining under a microscope for large, gram-positive pseudohyphae and spores (see p 155).
- Prescribe an oral suspension of nystatin (e.g., Mycostatin) 200,000 units for infants and 400,000–600,000 units for children and adults, gargled and swished in the mouth as long as possible before swallowing, four times a day, for at least two days beyond resolution of symptoms. Alternatively, prescribe clotrimazole in 10mg troches to be dissolved slowly in the mouth 5 times a day for 14 days.
- Look elsewhere for Candida: esophagitis, intertrigo, vaginitis, diaper rash, etc. All should respond to topical treatment with nystatin.

5

Pulmonary/Thoracic

Upper Respiratory Infection (Common Cold)

Presentation:

Most patients with colds do not visit emergency departments, unless they are unusually ill; the cold is prolonged more than a week, or it is progressing into bronchitis or serous otitis with new symptoms. The patient may want a note from a physician excusing him from work; or a prescription for antibiotics, which "seemed to help" the last time he had a cold.

The common denominator of URIs is inflammation of the respiratory mucosa. The nasal mucosa is usually red, swollen, and wet with reactive mucous. The pharynx is inflamed directly or secondarily to drainage of mucous from the nose, and swallowing may be painful (see p 75). Pharyngitis secondary to nasal drainage is typically worse upon arising in the morning, and signs and symptoms may be localized to the side that is dependent during sleep.

Occlusion of the ostia of paranasal sinuses permits buildup of mucous and pressure, leading to pain and predisposing bacterial superinfection (see p 73). Occlusion of the orifices of the eustachian tubes in the posterior pharynx permits imbalance of middle ear pressure and serous otitis (see p 62).

The larynx is also inflamed directly or secondarily to drainage of mucus, lowering the pitch and volume of the voice. The trachea can also be inflamed, producing coughing, and the bronchi can develop a bacterial superinfection. In addition to all these ills of the upper respiratory mucosa, there can be reactive lymphadenopathy of the anterior cervical chain, diffuse myalgias, and side effects of self-medication.

What to do:

- Perform a complete history and physical examination to document which of the above signs and symptoms are present; to rule out some other, underlying ailment; and to find any sign of

103

bacterial superinfection of ears, sinuses, pharynx, tonsils, epi-
glottis, bronchi, or lungs, that might require antibiotics or
other therapy.
- Explain the course of the viral illness, and the inadvisability of
indiscriminate antibiotics. Tailor drug treatment to the
patient's specific complaint as follows:
- For fever, headache, and myalgia, prescribe acetaminophen,
650mg q4h.
- To decongest the nose, ostia of sinuses, and eustachian tubes,
start with topical sympathomimetics (e.g., 0.5% phenylephrine
nose drops q4h, but only for 3 days) and add systemic sympathomimetics (pseudephedrine 60mg q6h or phenylpro-
panolamine 25mg q4h).
- To dry out a nose, or if the symptoms are probably caused by an
allergy, try antihistamines (e.g., chlorpheniramine 4mg q6h).
- To suppress coughing, prescribe dextromethorphan or codeine
10–20mg q6h.
- Arrange for followup if symptoms persist or worsen, or if new
problems develop.

What not to do:

- Do not get yourself bullied into inappropriate prescribing of
antibiotics. Most colds are self-limiting illnesses, and many
treatments may appear to work by coincidence alone. Your
suspicion that if you do not prescribe antibiotics, the insistent
patient will obtain them elsewhere is not justification for poor
medical practice.
- Do not undertake expensive diagnostic testing on uncomplicated cases.

Discussion:

Colds are produced by over a hundred different adeno and rhi-
noviruses, and influenza, coxsackie, and measles can also present as
a URI. Especially during the winter, when colds are epidemic, it
certainly helps to keep abreast of what is "going around," so that
you can intelligently advise patients on incubation periods, con-
tagiousness, expected symptoms, and duration; and also be able to
pick an unusual syndrome out of the background.
   The medications recommended here are available in various
combinations by prescription and over the counter. When is more
than symptomatic treatment indicated? Bacterial superinfections
require antibiotics. Mycoplasma pneumonia can present with
headache, cough, myalgias, and perhaps bullous myringitis, and
may respond to erythromycin. Coughing can precede wheezing as
an early sign of asthma, and response to beta agonists and the-

ophylline helps make the diagnosis. Antibiotics have not turned out to be very useful for acute bronchitis, and vitamin C as prophylaxis for colds has also not done well in controlled trials.

Rib Fracture and Costochondral Separation

Presentation:

A patient with an isolated rib fracture or a minor costochondral separation usually has a history of having fallen on the side of his chest. The initial chest pain may subside, but over the next few hours or days the pleuritic pain increases, interfering with sleep and activity and becoming severe with coughing or deep inspiration. The patient is often worried about having a broken rib.

Breath sounds bilaterally should be normal unless there is substantial splinting or a pneumothorax or hemothorax is present. There is point tenderness over the site of the injury and occasionally bony crepitance can be felt.

What to do:

- Check for pain with indirect stress on the suspected fracture site. Compress the rib medially if a posterior or anterior fracture is suspected. Compress the rib anteriorly/posteriorly if a fracture is suspected at a lateral location. When pain occurs at the suspected fracture site with indirect stress, this is clinical evidence of a fracture or separation and should be so documented on the chart.
- Examine the patient for possible associated injuries; e.g., do an abdominal exam to look for any signs of a splenic or hepatic injury.
- Obtain any history of chronic pulmonary problems or heavy smoking.
- Unless the patient is elderly or has pulmonary disease, have him try out a rib belt during his wait for x rays.
- Send the patient for a chest x ray to rule out a pneumothorax, hemothorax, evidence of pulmonary contusion, etc. Ordering rib films for radiological documentation of a fracture is optional.

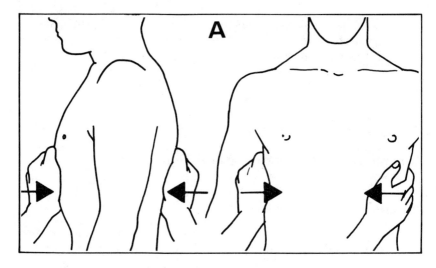

- When there is clinical or radiologic evidence of a rib fracture or chondral separation:
  a) Provide a potent oral analgesic (e.g., Tylenol with codeine, Percodan).
  b) Instruct the patient on the intermittent use of an elastic and velcro rib belt if reduces pain.
  c) Instruct the patient on the importance of deep breathing and coughing (using a pillow splint) to help prevent pneumonia. Tell him to take enough pain medicine to allow coughing and deep breathing.
  d) Provide the patient with an appropriate work excuse and refer him for followup care. Tell him to expect gradually decreasing discomfort for about two weeks, and forbid strenuous activity for approximately eight weeks.
- When there is no clinical or radiologic evidence of a fracture, treat the pain as you would any other contusion, using an appropriate analgesic.
- When multiple fractures or other injury which might compromise respiratory dynamics are present (especially in the elderly), hospitalization should be considered. Blood gases and pulmonary function tests can aid evaluation of breathing.

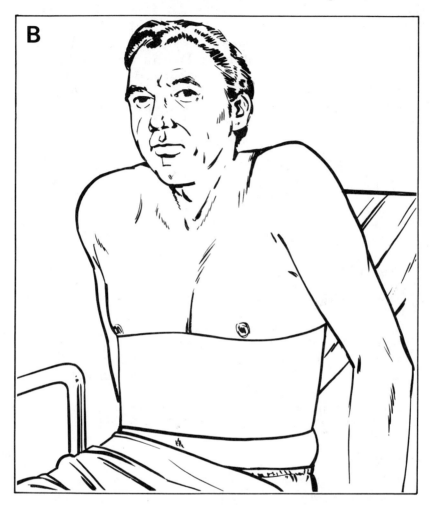

What not to do:

- Do not confuse simple rib fractures with massive blunt trauma to the chest. The evaluation and management is quite different.
- Do not tape ribs or use continuous strapping. This will lead to an atelectatic lung prone to developing pneumonia.
- Do not assume there is no fracture just because the x rays are negative. Rib fractures are often not apparent on x ray, especially when they occur in the cartilagenous portion of the rib. The patient deserves the disability period and analgesics commensurate with the real injury.

Discussion:

In the presence of severe pain one should consider the use of an intercostal nerve block or injection of the fracture hematoma with 0.5% bupivacaine hydrochloride (Marcaine). Because of the risks of pneumothorax or hemothorax, this procedure, in most cases, should be reserved for secondary management when initial treatment has proven ineffective.

Costochondritis

Presentation:

The patient's age is usually in the mid-teens through the thirties, and he complains of a day or more of dull, steady chest pain, perhaps following exertion, localized to the left or right of the sternum, without radiation, but worse with breathing and changes of position. He may be concerned about the possibility of a heart attack (though he may not voice his fear) but there is no associated nausea, vomiting, diaphoresis, or dyspnea.

The costal cartilages (connecting ribs to sternum) are tender to palpation, but the rest of the physical examination is normal.

What to do:

- Perform a thorough history and physical examination. Look for pleural or pericardial rubs, and obtain a cardiogram and chest x ray when there is any suspicion of a cardiac or pulmonary disorder. The presence of costochondritis does not exclude the possibility of myocardial infarction, pericarditis, pneumothorax, pneumonia, or pleural effusion.
- If there is no evidence of other disease, prescribe antiinflammatory analgesics (e.g., Motrin, Indocin), explain the condition and the lack of other disease, and instruct the patient to seek followup if symptoms have not improved in 1 to 2 days.

What not to do:

- Do not rule out myocardial infarction especially in the older patient, simply because there is tenderness over the costal cartilage, which could represent a coincidental finding, skin hypesthesia or contiguous inflammation secondary to the infarct.

Discussion:

This local inflammatory process is probably related to minor trauma, and would not be brought to medical attention so often if it did not resemble the pain of a heart attack. Careful reassurance of the patient is therefore most important. When exquisite tenderness localizes over the xyphoid cartilage this represents a xyphoiditis and can often be treated immediately with an injection of Depo-Medrol 40mg along with 5cc of 1% Xylocaine. (See below.)

Xyphoiditis

Presentation:

Patients are usually worried about having a heart attack. They complain about a lower substernal aching sensation that may spread across the anterior chest but should not radiate down the arms or into the jaw. They should not be diaphoretic, nauseated, or short of breath; but pain may worsen with deep inspiration or bending forward.

The pathognomonic finding during an otherwise normal physical exam is the exquisitely tender xyphoid cartilage that, upon palpation, elicits the pain of the chief complaint.

What to do:

- If one or more cardiac risk factors are present, or you are suspicious for any reason, get an ECG. This may also be necessary in order to adequately reassure the patient.
- In the event of fever or other positive physical findings relating to the chest, obtain a chest x ray.
- For mild symptoms, prescribe an antiinflammatory analgesic (e.g., naproxen sodium (Anaprox) 2 tabs at once then one every 6 hours). Warm, moist compresses may also be comforting.
- For more severe pain, inject the entire surface of the xyphoid cartilage with 4–5ccs of 1% lidocaine (Xylocaine) with epinephrine 1:10,000 mixed with 1cc (40mg) of methylprednisolone acetate suspension (Depo-Medrol). If this procedure makes the patient completely asymptomatic, then it provides you with a definitive diagnosis.

What not to do:

- Do not ignore cardiac symptoms in the presence of a tender xyphoid cartilage. The two conditions can occur simultaneously, and you obviously do not want to discharge the patient with an acute myocardial infarction.
- Do not forget to reassure the patient that his symptoms are not an indication of a heart attack but only a mild "arthritis-like" inflammation that may have been caused by a virus or minor trauma.

Discussion:

Injection of the xyphoid cartilage is similar to that of other trigger points (see p 168). Use a fine needle and fan out around the point of maximum tenderness. While injecting the xyphoid, you must use some caution to avoid entering the pleural cavity and causing a pneumothorax or injecting the myocardium by going beneath the xyphoid cartilage.

Tear Gas Exposure

Presentation:

The patient may have been in a riot dispersed by the police, or accidently sprayed by his own can of Mace. He complains of burning of the eyes, nose, mouth, and skin; tearing and inability to open eyes because of the severe stinging; sneezing, coughing, a runny nose, and perhaps nausea, vomiting, and abdominal pains. These signs and symptoms last for 15–30 minutes after exposure.

What to do:

- Segregate victims lest they contaminate others. Medical personnel should don gowns, gloves, and masks, and help victims remove contaminated clothes and/or shower with soap and water to remove tear gas from their skin.
- If eye pain lasts longer than 15–20 minutes, examine with fluorescein for corneal erosions, which may be produced by tear gas.
- Look for signs of, and warn patient about, allergic reactions to tear gas, including bronchospasm and contact dermatitis.

What not to do:

- Do not rush to help or allow other helpers to rush in heedlessly and themselves become incapacitated.

Discussion:

Agents commonly used as tear gas include CN or Mace, which is sprayed in a weak water solution, CS which is burned, and produces symptoms as long as the victim is in the smoke, and CR which is more potent and longer lasting.

Inhalation Injury

Presentation:

The patient was trapped in an enclosed space for some time with toxic gas or fumes produced by a fire, leak, evaporation of solvent, chemical reaction, fermentation of silage, etc., and comes to the ED complaining of some combination of coughing, wheezing, shortness of breath, irritation or running of eyes or nose, chest or abdominal pain, or skin irritation. Symptoms may develop immediately or after a lag of as much as a day. On physical examination, the victim may smell of the agent or be covered with soot or burns. Inflammation of the eyes, nose, mouth, or upper airway may be visible, while pulmonary irritation may be evident as coughing, ronchi, rales, or wheezing, although these signs may also take up to a day to develop.

What to do:

- Separate the victim from the toxic agent—e.g., removing clothes, hosing down, or showering with soap and water.
- Make sure the victim is breathing adequately, and then add oxygen at 6 to 12 liters per minute. Oxygen helps most inhalation injuries, and is essential in treating carbon monoxide poisoning.
- Look for evidence that may help identify the exposure: was there a fire? what was burning? was there an associated blast? what material is on the victim? what does he smell of? what are his current signs and symptoms? is there soot in the posterior pharynx? there may be evidence of a specific toxin which calls for a specific antidote (e.g., muscle fasiculations, small pupils, and wet lungs may imply organophosphates which should be treated with atropine).

- Unless the patient is asymptomatic, obtain a chest x ray and arterial blood gases (record the rate of O_2 being administered). An increased alveolar-arterial PO_2 difference may be the earliest sign of pulmonary injury; but even if the CXR and ABGs are normal, they can serve as a baseline for evaluation of later pulmonary problems. Strongly consider obtaining a carboxyhemoglobin (COHgb) level, if only as a marker of other combustion products.
- If the patient has difficulty breathing or any x ray or blood gas abnormality suggesting acute pulmonary injury, he should be kept on oxygen and admitted to the hospital, even if only overnight. Wheezing and bronchospasm may be allergic reactions and respond to conventional doses of aminophylline (5mg/kg iv over 20 minutes); but, if not promptly reversible, are probably a sign of pulmonary injury.
- If there are no signs or symptoms of inhalation injury (or all have resolved) in one hour, it may be safe to send the patient home, with instructions to return for reevaluation the next day, or sooner if any pulmonary signs or symptoms occur (e.g., coughing, wheezing, shortness of breath).
- Repeat vital signs, physical exam, ABGs, and CXR in 12 to 24 hours, looking for any changes indicative of late pulmonary injury.

What not to do:

- Do not assume the patient is all right following an inhalation injury simply because there are no symptoms and no ABG or CXR abnormalities evident in the first few hours. Some agents produce pulmonary inflammation which develops over 12 to 24 hours.
- Do not wait for carboxyhemoglobin levels before giving 100% O_2 for suspected carbon monoxide poisoning. Begin O_2 as soon as possible. One hundred percent oxygen (which requires a tight-fitting mask and a reservoir for administration) will reduce the half-life of carboxyhemoglobin from six hours to 1½ hours.
- Do not insist on having the patient breathe room air for a period before obtaining ABGs. If the O_2 is helping, its withdrawal is a disservice, and the alveolar-arterial O_2 gradient can still be estimated with a high concentration of inspired oxygen.

Discussion:

One category of inhalation injury is caused by relatively inert gases, such as carbon dioxide and fuel gases (e.g., methane, ethane, propane, acetylene) which displace air and oxygen, producing asphyxia. Treatment consists of removing the victim from the gas and allowing him to breathe air or oxygen, and attending to any damage caused by the period of hypoxia (e.g., myocardial infarction, cerebral injury).

A second category of inhalation injury is from irritants, such as (in roughly decreasing order of solubility in water) ammonia, formaldehyde, chloramine (NH_2Cl), chlorine, nitrogen dioxide and phosgene ($COCl_2$) which, when dissolved in the water lining the respiratory mucosa, produce a chemical burn and an inflammatory response. The first few listed, being more soluble, tend to produce more upper airway burns (also irritating eyes, nose, and mouth) while the latter gases listed, being less water soluble, produce greater pulmonary injury and respiratory distress syndrome.

A third category of inhalation injury includes inhaled agents which are systemic toxins, such as carbon monoxide, hydrogen cyanide, and hydrogen sulfide, (all of which interfere with the delivery of oxygen for cellular energy production) and aromatic and halogenated hydrocarbons (which can produce liver, kidney, brain, lung, and other organ damage).

A final category of inhalation injury is allergic, in which inhaled gases, particles or aerosols produce bronchospasm and edema, much like asthma or spasmodic croup.

6

Gastrointestinal

Singultus (Hiccups)

Presentation:

Recurring, unpredictable, clonic contractions of the diaphragm produce sharp inhalations. Hiccups are usually precipitated by some combination of laughing, talking, eating, and drinking, but may also occur spontaneously. Most cases also resolve spontaneously, and do not come to the emergency department unless prolonged or severe.

What to do:

- Stimulate the patient's soft palate by rubbing it with a swab, catheter tip or finger, just short of stimulating a gag reflex, and continue this for a few minutes. Alternatively, you may stimulate the same general area by depositing a tablespoon of granulated sugar at the base of the tongue, in the area of the lingual tonsils, and letting it dissolve. Such maneuvers (or their placebo effect) may abolish simple cases of hiccups.
- If hiccups continue, look for a cause, and ask about precipitating factors. Look in the ears (foreign bodies against the tympanic membrane can cause hiccups). Examine the chest and abdomen, perhaps including upright chest x rays, to look for processes irritating the phrenic nerve or diaphragm. Perform a neurological exam, looking for evidence of partial continuous seizures or brainstem lesions.
- If hiccups persist, try chlorpromazine (Thorazine) 25–50mg tid or qid. (The same dose may be given im.) Arrange for followup and additional evaluation.

Discussion:

The common denominator among various hiccup cures seems to be stimulation of the glossopharyngeal nerve, but, as for every self-limiting disease, there are always many effective cures.

Esophageal Food Bolus Obstruction (Steakhouse Syndrome)

Presentation:

The patient will develop symptoms immediately after swallowing a large bolus of food. Usually this bolus is made of inadequately chewed meat, the result of wearing dentures or being too embarrassed to spit out a large piece of gristle. The patient often develops substernal chest pain that may mimic the pain of a myocardial infarction. This discomfort though, is followed by retained salivary secretions and, unlike infarction, leads to drooling. The patient is usually found with a receptacle under his mouth into which he is repeatedly spitting. At times these secretions will cause paroxysms of coughing, gagging, or choking.

What to do:

- Insert a small N.G. tube to the point of obstruction and attach it to low intermittent suction, to assist the patient in handling excess secretions and reduce the risk of aspiration.
- A barium swallow can be done to confirm the diagnosis and localize the level of obstruction. When classic symptoms are present and there is no sign of any complication, this procedure can be deferred.
- Give 1 unit of glucagon iv to decrease lower esophageal sphincter pressure. This will sometimes allow for passage of a food bolus. If there is no response repeat after 30 minutes.
- If the food does not pass spontaneously, prepare the patient for manual extraction. Start an intravenous line for drug administration and anesthetize the pharynx with Cetacaine spray or viscous lidocaine 2%. Place the patient on his side and slowly administer diazepam (Valium) intravenously until the patient is very drowsy. Take a gastric Ewald lavage tube, cut off the end until there are no side ports and round off the new tip with scissors. Push the Ewald tube through the patient's mouth until

the obstruction is reached. Take a large aspiration syringe, have an assistant apply suction to the free end of the Ewald tube and slowly withdraw it. If suction is maintained, the bolus will come up with the tubing.

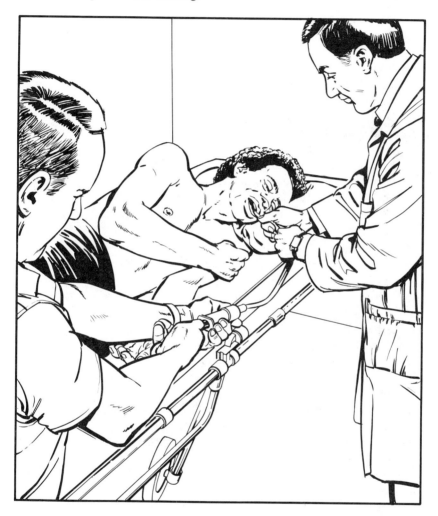

- If the patient is unable to tolerate this procedure or you are unsuccessful in removing the foreign body, consult with an endoscopist for an early removal with a flexible fiberoptic esophagoscope.
- When removal of the food bolus has been successful, early medical followup should be provided for a comprehensive evaluation of the esophagus. Patients who have experienced a prolonged obstruction or do not have complete resolution of all

their symptoms should be admitted to the hospital for further observation and management.

What not to do:

- Do not try to force the food bolus down with the Ewald tube or any other catheter or dilator. This may cause an esophageal tear or perforation.
- Do not use oral enzymes such as papain, trypsin or chymotrypsin. This treatment is slow, ineffective, and may possibly carry a risk of enzyme-induced esophageal perforation.
- Do not attempt to remove a hard, sharp, esophageal foreign body using any of the above techniques. This very likely will cause an esophageal injury.
- Do not count on watchful waiting to resolve the patient's problem. Prolonged delay may lead to local esophageal ischemia and the potential risk of subsequent perforation.

Discussion:

Patients who experience a food bolus obstruction of the esophagus often have an underlying structural lesion. One of the more common lesions is a benign stricture secondary to reflux esophagitis. Another abnormality, the classic Schatzki's ring (distal esophageal mucosal ring), especially above a hiatal hernia, may present with the "steakhouse syndrome" in which obstruction occurs and is relieved spontaneously. Other associated problems include postoperative narrowing, neoplasms and cervical webs as well as motility disorders, neurological disease and collagen vascular disease.

Additional modes of therapy include the use of sublingual nitroglycerin, or nifedipine (not usually as effective as intravenous glucagon) and the oral administration of tartaric acid and sodium bicarbonate.

This last technique is of uncertain safety and utilizes 15ml of tartaric acid (18.7g/100ml) followed immediately by 15ml of sodium bicarbonate (10g/100ml). Carbon dioxide is formed and, with the upper esophageal sphincter closed, the increased pressure distends the esophagus and forces the bolus into the stomach. Retching will occur and although no complications have been reported with this technique, it is recommended that it not be used when the obstruction has been prolonged.

Swallowed Foreign Body

Presentation:

Parents bring in a young child shortly after he has swallowed a coin, safety pin, toy, etc. Disturbed patients may present themselves to the hospital on repeated occasions, at times accumulating a sizeable load of ingested material.

What to do:

- Ask about symptoms and examine the patient, looking for signs of airway obstruction (e.g., coughing, wheezing) or bowel obstruction or perforation (vomiting, melena, abdominal pain, abnormal bowel sounds).
- Obtain 2 plain x ray views of throat to at least the mid abdomen to determine if indeed anything was ingested or if the FB has become lodged someplace or produced an obstruction. A barium swallow may occasionally be necessary to locate a nonopaque FB in the esophagus.
- An FB lodged in the esophagus for more than a day should be removed endoscopically, because it is likely to cause a problem, and is still accessible. An alternate approach to endoscopy is to pass a small Foley catheter fluoroscopically past the foreign body, inflate the balloon and draw it back. The patient should be placed on his side in the Trendelenburg position to reduce the risk of aspiration.
- When an FB has passed into the stomach and there are no symptoms which demand immediate removal, discharge the patient with instructions to return for reevaluation in 2–3 days (or sooner if he develops nausea, vomiting, abdominal pain, rectal pain, or rectal bleeding). Having parents sift through stools is often unproductive (one missed stool negates days of hard work).

What not to do:

- Do not use ipecac for foreign body ingestions. Emesis is effective for emptying the stomach of liquid and dissolved drugs, but not for removing FBs from the esophagus.
- Do not automatically assume that an ingested FB should be surgically removed. The vast majority of potentially injurious FBs pass through the alimentary tract without mishap. Operate only when the patient is actually being harmed by the swallowed FB.
- Do not attempt to push an FB down the esophagus with a nasogastric tube or other such device.

Discussion:

The narrowest strait in the gastrointestinal tract is usually the cricopharyngeus muscle at the level of the thyroid cartilage. Next narrowest is usually the pylorus, followed by the lower esophageal sphincter and the ileocecal valve. Thus, anything which passes the throat will probably pass through the anus as well.

In general, FBs below the diaphragm should be left alone. A swallowed FB can irritate or perforate the GI tract anywhere, but does not require treatment until complications occur. Even safety pins and razor blades usually pass without incident.

Large button batteries (the size of quarters) have become stuck in the esophagus, eroded through the esophageal wall, and produced a fatal exsanguination; but the smaller variety, and batteries which passed into the gut, have not been such a danger.

Innocuous Ingestions

Presentation:

Frightened parents call or arrive in the emergency room with a two-year-old child who has just swallowed some household product.

What to do:

- Establish exactly what was ingested (have them locate the container or bring in a sample if possible), how much, how long ago, as well as any symptoms and treatment so far.
- If there is any question about the substance, its toxicity, or its treatment, call the regional poison control center. In fact, it is a good policy to call the regional poison center even if you are completely comfortable managing the case, so that they can record the ingestion for epidemiologic purposes.
- If there is any question of this being a toxic ingestion, give the child syrup of ipecac, 15ml po, followed by one glass of water, and expect to see emesis in 20–40 minutes.
- Reassure the parents and child, and instruct them to call or return to the ED if there are any problems. Teach parents how to keep all poisons beyond the reach of children; how to get syrup of ipecac (at any pharmacy, without a prescription, for $1–$2) for home use and how to call the regional poison center first for any future ingestions.

What not to do:

- Do not totally believe what you're told about the nature of the ingestion. Often some of the information immediately available is wrong. Suspect the worst.
- Do not depend on product labels to give you accurate information on toxicity. Some lethal poisons carry warnings no more serious than "use as directed," or "for external use only."
- Do not follow the instructions on the package regarding what to do if a product is ingested. These are often inaccurate or out-of-date.
- Do not give ipecac for emesis of liquids that are corrosive or toxic only when aspirated, such as hydrocarbons.
- Do not improvise treatment of a patient referred to you by the regional poison center. They probably have special information and a treatment plan to share with you, if they have not called already.

Discussion:

Fortunately, most products designed to be played with by children are also designed to be non-toxic when ingested. This includes chalk, crayons, ink, paste, paint, and Play-Doh. Many drugs, such as birth control pills and thyroid hormone, are relatively non-toxic, as are most laundry bleaches, the mercury in thermometers and many plants. On the other hand, some apparently innocuous household products are surprisingly toxic, including camphorated oil, cigarettes, dishwasher soap, oil of wintergreen, and vitamins with iron.

Because both the ingredients of common products and the treatment of ingestions continue to change, broad statements and lists are not reliable. **Your best strategy is always to call the regional poison control center. See Appendix, p 287 for a list.**

Food Poisoning—Staphylococcal

Presentation:

The patient is brought to the ED 1 to 6 hours after eating, with severe nausea, vomiting, and abdominal cramps progressing into diarrhea. He appears very ill—pale, diaphoretic, tachycardic, orthostatic, perhaps complaining of paresthesias or feeling as if he is "going to die." Others may have similar symptoms from eating the same food.

The physical examination, however, is reassuring. There is minimal abdominal tenderness, localized, if at all, to the epigastrium or to the rectus abdominus muscle (which is strained by the vomiting).

What to do:

- Completely examine the patient, and perform any tests needed to rule out myocardial infarction, perforated ulcer, dissecting aneurysm, or any of the catastrophes which can present in similar fashion.
- In the meantime, infuse Ringer's lactate iv and observe the patient, doing repeated vital sign checks and physical examination. In younger patients, who have the renal and cardiovascular reserve to handle rapid hydration, 1–2 liters infused over as many hours often provides dramatic improvement in all symptoms.
- If the patient is improving, and beginning to tolerate oral fluids, discharge him with instructions to advance his diet gradually over the next day, starting with clear liquids, crackers, and toast. He should expect to be eating and feeling well in another 1 or 2 days.
- If symptoms resolve more slowly, you may want to discharge the patient with a single dose of an antiemetic or antispasmotic for comfort.
- If hypotension or other significant symptoms persist; if the patient cannot tolerate parenteral rehydration, or cannot resume oral intake; he may have to be admitted.

What not to do:

- Do not immediately resort to medications (e.g., Compazine, Tigan) for nausea and vomiting. They may interfere with elimination of toxins, and do not help correct the fluid and electrolyte imbalances responsible for many of the symptoms.
- Do not immediately resort to medications (e.g., Lomotil, Imodium) for cramping and diarrhea, for the same reasons.
- Do not skimp on intravenous fluids.
- Do not pursue expensive laboratory investigations on straightforward cases.
- Do not presume food poisoning without a good history for it.

Discussion:

Many of the symptoms accompanying any gastroenteritis seem to be related to electrolyte disturbances and dehydration, which can be substantial even in the absence of copious vomiting and diarrhea, and resistant to oral rehydration, because the gut is unable to absorb, and allows liter after liter to pool in its lumen. Lactated Ringer's solution is the choice for intravenous rehydration, because it approximates normal serum electrolytes, and can be infused rapidly.

The most common food poisoning seen in most EDs is caused by the heat-stable toxin of Staphylococcus, which is introduced into food from infections on handlers, and grows when the food sits warm. Chemical toxins have a similar presentation, but the onset of symptoms may be more immediate. Other bacterial food poisonings usually present with onset of symptoms later than 1–6 hours after eating, less nausea and vomiting, more cramping and diarrhea, and longer courses. A clearly implicated food source may give a clue to the etiology: shellfish suggesting *Vibrio parahemolyticus*, rice suggesting *Bacillus cereus*, and meat or eggs suggesting *Staphylococcus, Clostridium, Salmonella, E. Coli,* etc.

Whenever someone suffers any gastrointestinal upset, it is natural, if not instinctive, to implicate the last food eaten. Caution patients (especially if they are planning to sue the food supplier) that the diagnosis of food poisoning cannot be established without a group outbreak or a sample of tainted food for analysis.

Diarrhea

Presentation:

Complaints may range from acute, copious diarrhea producing shock, to concern because an occasional stool is not well formed. Typically, there is crampy pain throughout the abdomen, especially before a diarrhea stool, and some irritation of the anus. Tenesmus (the frequent urge to defecate) can exist without diarrhea.

What to do:

- Ask specifically about the frequency of stools, the volume (much liquid implies a defect in absorption in the small bowel, while tenesmus producing little more than mucus implies inflammation of the rectosigmoid wall), the character (color, odor, blood, or mucus) and the consistency (like water or just loose stool). Ask about travel, medications (including antibiotics), prior similar symptoms, and nocturnal symptoms (rare with functional disease).

- Perform orthostatic vital signs and urinalysis and weigh pediatric patients. Any symptoms, fall in pressure, or pulse rise of more than 10–20 after one minute of standing suggest hypovolemia. A urine specific gravity over 1.020 also suggests hypovolemia, and ketones of 2+ or greater suggest starvation ketosis.
- Perform a rectal exam and obtain a sample of stool for Wright's or Gram stain. (If the rectal ampulla is empty, wait until the patient has another stool.) If there are any white cells in 5 oil-immersion fields, assume the problem is invasive or inflammatory (e.g., Salmonella, Shigella, Campylobacter, Entameba, or ulcerative colitis). If no white blood cells are visible, assume the diarrhea is due to virus or toxin.
- Patients with invasive processes (WBC in diarrhea stool) should have stool cultured and followup arranged for reevaluation, reculture and perhaps, examinations for parasites as well.
- Patients with viral or toxic diarrhea (no stool WBCs) may need followup only if they have continued diarrhea, abdominal pain and/or fever.
- Both classes of diarrhea are best treated with absorbent bulk laxatives, such as ground psyllium seeds (Metamucil), 1 tbsp in a glass of water up to qid (with meals and at bedtime).
- To adsorb toxins and provide some binding effect, you can add Amphojel, or Kaopectate, also one tbsp qid, to the Metamucil. Alternatively, you can start bismuth subsalicylate (Pepto-Bismol), two tablespoonsful every half hour until symptoms subside, or a total of eight doses are taken. Pepto-Bismol has also been demonstrated very effective in toxin-mediated diarrhea, but this preparation does contain salicylates, and bismuth will turn stools black.
- Patients with severe dehydration that cannot be reversed orally require intravenous fluids, and, if there are other severe complications, may have to be admitted to hospital, perhaps on infectious isolation precautions.

What not to do:

- Do not routinely use narcotics to paralyze peristalsis. Lomotil, Paregoric, Imodium, etc., will reduce cramps and frequency of diarrhea; but they may slow elimination of toxins or organisms, have little effect on the electrolyte imbalance symptoms; and might even potentiate bowel perforation in invasive conditions like salmonella, amebic dysentery, and ulcerative colitis.
- Do not omit the rectal exam, which may disclose a fecal impaction or any abscess.

Discussion:

When you prescribe Metamucil, patients may remind you that they have diarrhea, not constipation. Explain that an agent absorbing water in the gut lumen relieves both problems, and obviates rebound constipation often produced by narcotics and binders used for diarrhea.

Most bacterial diarrheas do not require treatment with antibiotics, which can even prolong the illness or produce a carrier state. Camphylobacter (currently the most common cause of bacterial diarrhea in the U.S.) is usually treated with oral erythromycin, and Shigella is usually treated with oral trimethoprim—sulfamethoxazole (Bactrim or Septra). Unfortunately, the responsible organism is difficult to identify on clinical grounds, and the best strategy usually is to await culture results.

Infants can become severely dehydrated in short order with viral diarrhea, while the old patients medicated for pain or psychosis can develop chronic constipation and fecal impaction, which can also present as diarrhea. Promiscuous homosexual men can spread unusual enteric infections via anal sex.

Irritable bowel syndrome, food allergies, lactose intolerance, and parasite infestation can produce relapsing diarrhea, which may require followup to establish the symptom pattern and diagnosis.

Gas Pain and Constipation

Presentation:

Excruciating, sharp, crampy, migratory abdominal pain may double the patient over, but lasts only a few seconds and is relieved by bowel movement and passing flatus. It may be related to loud bowel sounds (or borborygmi) but not to position, eating, or other causes, and is not accompanied by other symptoms, such as nausea, vomiting, diarrhea, urinary urgency, etc. Rarely are patients awakened with nocturnal symptoms. The physical examination is also benign, with no tenderness, masses, organomegaly, or other abnormalities. Bowel sounds, however, may become loud during each episode of cramps.

What to do:

• Take a thorough history and perform a complete physical

examination, including rectal and/or pelvic examination, and a repeat abdominal examination after an interval.

- If the presentation is not clear, consider using diagnostic tests, like urinalysis (to help rule out renal colic or urinary tract infection); or differential white blood cell count (a clue to infection or inflammation).
- If constipation is part of the problem, disimpact the rectum, if necessary, and try one enema in the ED.
- Instruct the patient to try relieving symptoms with ambulation, and local heat, and to return to the ED or see his personal physician if symptoms do not resolve over the next 12–24 hours. Suggest bulk in the form of bran or Metamucil for prophylaxis.
- If the problem is chronic or recurrent, or associated with alternating constipation and diarrhea, suspect irritable colon, inflammatory bowel disease, and/or diverticulitis.

What not to do:

- Do not discharge the patient without one or two hours of observation, and two abdominal examinations. Many abdominal catastrophes may appear improved for short periods.

Enterobiasis (Pinworm or Threadworm)

Presentation:

The patient complains of perianal itching which is worse at night, and may contribute to insomnia or superinfection of the excoriated perianal skin. Often, an entire family is affected.

What to do:

- Examine the anus to rule out other causes of itching, such as rectal prolapse, fecal leakage, hemorrhoids, lice (pediculosis), fungal infections (tinea or candidiasis), or bacterial infections (erythrasma).
- Look for pinworms directly (especially if the patient comes in at night), and by pressing the sticky side of cellophane tape to the perianal skin. Examine the tape under the low power of the microscope for female worms, approximately 1cm long, 0.5mm in diameter, with pointed tails. (Use shiny rather than "invisible" tape, because the latter's rough surface makes microscopy difficult.)

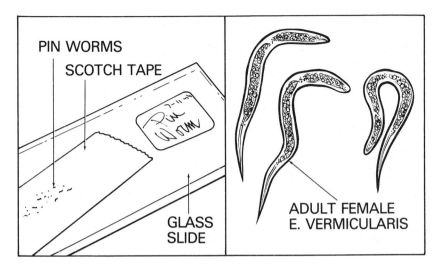

- If you see pinworms or still suspect them, administer a single oral dose of pyrantel pamoate 11mg/kg (maximum 1gm) to all family members (Antiminth oral suspension, 1ml/10lb). Alternate drugs include mebendazole and pyrvinium pamoate.
- Explain to all concerned that this is not a dangerous infection, and that it should be eradicated from the whole family after one treatment (which may be repeated in two or more weeks if there are recurrences).

Discussion:

Pinworms mostly live in the colon, and females migrate down to the perianal skin to lay eggs at night. Eggs on contaminated fingers re-enter via the mouth, but remain viable for several days on surfaces around the house. Perhaps 10% of the U.S. population harbors pinworms.

Hemorrhoids

Presentation:

The patient usually complains either of severe pain which is worse with sitting, defecating, or moving, or of bleeding, which is noticed on the toilet paper or dripping into the toilet bowl, but not actually mixed in with stools.

What to do:

- If the problem is rectal bleeding, it should be approached as any other GI bleeding. The amount of bleeding should be quantified with orthostatic vital signs and a hematocrit; the rectosigmoid should be examined with an anoscope or sigmoidoscope to look for bleeding from the colon; and, if there remains any question of bleeding from above, the stomach should be lavaged via a nasogastric tube.

- If the problem is pain, the rectum should be examined using a topical anesthetic (e.g., lidocaine jelly) as a lubricant. First look for thrombosed external hemorrhoids and prolapsed internal hemorrhoids. Have the patient perform a Valsalva maneuver as you provide traction on the skin of the buttocks, to evert the anus. Examine the posterior mucosa for anal fissures. After the topical anesthesia has taken effect, complete the digital rectal exam, looking for internal hemorrhoids and evidence of rectal abscesses or other masses.

- If topical anesthetics on the rectal mucosa help control the pain, provide for more of the same, perhaps also with some added corticosteroid for anti-inflammatory effect (e.g., Anusol-HC). Suppositories are convenient, if the patient can comfortably insert them; otherwise prescribe cream or foam (e.g., Proctofoam-HC, applied externally rather than internally).

- If a thrombosed external hemorrhoid is still quite painful, you may try injecting around it with a local anesthetic to allow for an adequate digital exam. If fresh (not organized or scarred) the

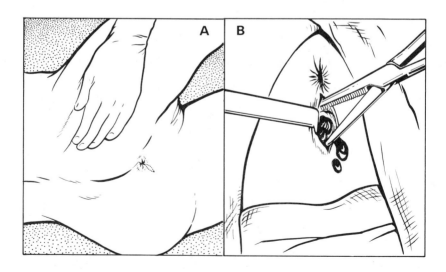

thrombus may extrude via an elliptical incision over the anal mucosa. Locular clots can be broken up by inserting a straight hemostat into the wound, and spreading the tips, thereby allowing the clots to be expressed. Pain relief from surgical technique can be dramatic, but this procedure may cause more pain than it cures, and sometimes produces bleeding.

- Instruct the patient to prevent constipation by using bulk laxatives (bran, Metamucil), treat lesser pain and itching with compresses, Tucks, and sitz baths, and arrange followup as needed.
- Small ulcerated hemorrhoids usually do not require any treatment for hemostasis. Bulk laxatives and gentle cleansing are generally all that is required.

What not to do:

- Do not labor to reduce prolapsed hemorrhoids unless they are part of a large rectal prolapse with some strangulation. You may increase the pain, and everything may prolapse again when the patient stands or strains.
- Do not traumatize the patient with your examination.
- Do not miss infectious and neoplastic processes which can resemble or coexist with hemorrhoids. Always provide appropriate followup for patients with rectal bleeding and/or pain.

Discussion:

The diagnosis of "hemorrhoids" may cover a variety of minor ailments of the anus, which may or may not be related to the hemorrhoidal veins. The ED approach consists of ruling out more serious problems, and then providing the patient with symptomatic relief.

Rectal Foreign Body

Presentation:

The typical patient is a male homosexual in his 30's or 40's. Rectal and/or lower abdominal pain may or may not be present. The object is generally inserted by the patient or a partner for sexual stimulation; then it causes pain, becomes irretrievable, or both.

When interviewed privately, the patient will usually give an accurate accounting of what happened. Often, however, outlandish explanations (such as having fallen onto the object) are proffered by the patient and at times a patient will not volunteer that any object has been inserted.

What to do:

- Perform an abdominal and rectal exam. If there are signs of peritoneal inflammation, such as rebound tenderness or pain with movement, a perforation of the bowel should be suspected. Start appropriate intravenous lines, draw blood for laboratory analysis and obtain flat and upright abdominal x rays to look for free air. Notify your surgical consultants at once.
- If there are no signs of perforation, obtain flat and upright abdominal films to help define the nature, size, and number of foreign objects, as well as to reveal unsuspected free air.
- Sedate the patient with meperidine (Demerol) and/or diazepam (Valium) to help in the removal of the FB. Place the patient on his side in the Sims position. If anal discomfort persists, locally infiltrate 1% lidocaine (Xylocaine).
- When the object can be reached by the examining finger and it is of a nature that will allow it to be grasped, the lax anal sphincters of many of these patients may allow you slowly to insert as much of your gloved hand as possible to grab the object and gradually extricate it.
- If you are unable to pull out the foreign body with your hand, there are a number of techniques that can be used to break the vacuum behind the object and get a purchase on it:
  a) Slide a large Foley catheter with a 30cc balloon past the object, inflate the balloon, and apply traction to the catheter. (This can be used in conjunction with any of the other techniques.)
  b) Under direct visualization with an anoscope or vaginal speculum, you can attempt to grasp the object with a tenaculum, sponge forcep, Kelly clamp or tonsil snare.
  c) An open object, like a jar or bottle, can be filled with wet plaster, into which a tongue blade can be inserted like a popsickle stick. When the plaster hardens, traction can be applied to the tongue blade.
  d) Forceps or soup spoons can be used to "deliver" a round object.
- With an object that is too high to reach, the patient can be admitted and sedated for removal the next day.
- When the object cannot be removed due to patient discomfort or sphincter tightness, then removal must be accomplished in the OR under spinal or general anesthesia.

- When blood is present in the rectum or the object was one capable of doing harm to the bowel, then sigmoidoscopy should be performed after removal of the foreign body. When pain persists or there is any lingering suspicion of a bowel perforation, keep the patient for observation.

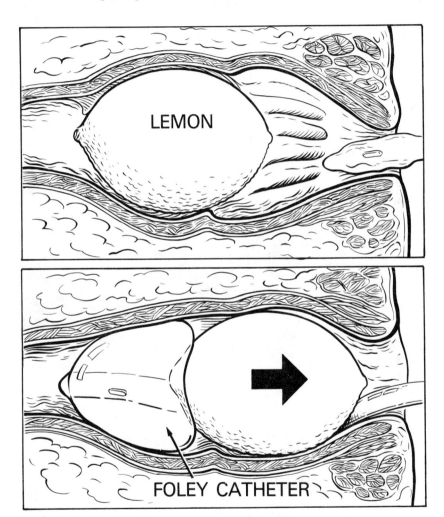

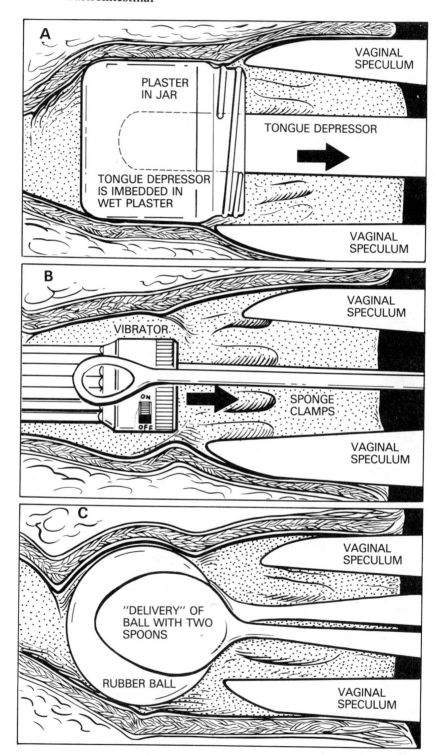

A

VAGINAL
SPECULUM

PLASTER
IN JAR

TONGUE DEPRESSOR

TONGUE DEPRESSOR
IS IMBEDDED IN
WET PLASTER

VAGINAL
SPECULUM

B

VAGINAL
SPECULUM

VIBRATOR

SPONGE
CLAMPS

VAGINAL
SPECULUM

C

VAGINAL
SPECULUM

"DELIVERY" OF
BALL WITH TWO
SPOONS

RUBBER BALL

VAGINAL
SPECULUM

What not to do:

- Do not pressure the patient into giving you an accurate story. He often is embarrassed or worried about what you will think of him. Your intimidation will not help.
- Do not push the object higher into the colon while attempting to remove it.
- Do not blindly grab for an object with a tenaculum or other such device. This can itself lead to a perforation.
- Do not attempt to remove sharp, jagged objects such as broken glass via the rectum. These should only be removed under anesthesia in the OR.
- Do not send a patient who is having continued pain home. Admit him and observe for peritoneal signs, increased pain, fever, and a rising white count.

Discussion:

Most rectal foreign bodies (e.g., vibrators, dildos, broom handles, bottles, lightbulbs, balls, fruits, and vegetables) can be removed safely in the emergency department. Some practitioners quite reasonably forego x rays prior to manipulation if the patient is free of pain and fever.

7

Urologic

Lower Urinary Tract Infection (Cystitis)

Presentation:

The patient (usually female) complains of urinary frequency and urgency, dysuria, and suprapubic pain. There may have been some antecedent trauma (e.g., sexual intercourse) to inoculate the bladder, and there may be blood in the urine (hemorrhagic cystitis).

Usually, there is *no* labial irritation or vaginal discharge (which would suggest vaginitis); or fever, chills, nausea, flank pain, or costovertebral angle tenderness (which would suggest an upper urinary tract infection.)

What to do:

- If available in the ED, dip stick for white cells or Gram stain a sample of urine. The presence of any white cells in a clean specimen on microscopic examination confirms the infection, gram-positive cocci suggest an enterococcal (group D Strep) infection for which ampicillin or amoxicillin would be the preferred antibiotic.
- If the clinical picture is clearly that of a lower UTI, give a single oral dose of amoxicillin 3gm, sulfasoxazole 2gm, or trimethoprim 160–320mg plus sulfamethoxazole 800–1600mg (Bactrim or Septra, one to two double strength tablets). Instruct the patient to drink plenty of liquids (such as cranberry juice) but do not push fluids when treating children or adult males.
- If the dysuria is severe, you may also prescribe Pyridium, 200mg tid for 2 days only, to act as a surface anesthetic in the bladder. Warn the patient that it will stain her urine (and perhaps clothes) orange.

- Arrange for followup in 2 days if the symptoms have not completely resolved. If necessary, urine culture and a longer course of antibiotics can be undertaken then.

What not to do:

- Do not undertake expensive urine cultures for every straightforward lower urinary tract infection.
- Do not follow the single-dose regimen for a possible upper urinary tract infection.
- Do not give probenecid with the single dose of antibiotic. Probenecid is used in the single-dose treatment of gonorrhea, *to block excretion* of antibiotic into the urine and sustain high plasma levels, but here the entire point is *to excrete* the antibiotic into the urine.

Discussion:

Previous medical practice was to prescribe a 7–14 day course of antibiotics for uncomplicated UTIs, but recent studies have shown that shorter courses (including a single dose) are just as efficacious.

If there is any doubt about the diagnosis, a formal urinalysis can provide valuable information. In a clean sediment (free of epithelial cells) one white cell per 400x field suggests a significant pyuria, although clinicians accustomed to imperfect samples usually set a threshold of 3–5 WBCs per field. In addition, Trichomonas may be appreciated swimming in the urinary sediment, indicating a different etiology for urinary symptoms or associated vaginitis.

In a straightforward lower UTI, urine culture may be reserved for cases which fail to resolve with single-dose therapy. In complicated or doubtful cases, however, or with recurrences, a urine culture before initial treatment may be helpful.

Healthy women may be expected to suffer a few episodes of lower urinary tract infection in a lifetime without indicating any major structural problem, but recurrences at short intervals suggest inadequate treatment or underlying abnormalities. Men, however, who have longer urethras and far fewer lower UTIs, probably should be evaluated urologically after just one episode.

Upper Urinary Tract Infection (Pyelonephritis)

Presentation:

The patient has some combination of urinary frequency, urgency, dysuria, flank pain, nausea, fever, and chills. On physical examination, there is tenderness elicited by percussing the costovertebral angle over the kidneys. The urinalysis may help establish the diagnosis with tubular casts of white cells.

What to do:

- Examine urine for presence of gram-positive cocci (presumptively enterococci) or the more usual gram-negative rods, and send for culture and sensitivity.
- If the patient appears toxic, with a high fever or white count, nausea or vomiting to prevent adequate oral medication and hydration, or any sign of urinary obstruction or developing sepsis, he or she should be admitted to the hospital for intravenous antibiotics.
- For the majority of stable patients, oral hydration and antibiotics will be sufficient (e.g., sulfamethoxazole 2gm initially, then 1gm tid x 10d, or trimethoprim 160mg/sulfamethoxazole 800mg qid x 10d). For suspected enterococci, amoxicillin 500mg tid may be better.
- Arrange definite followup for reculture and reexamination in 10 days. Have the patient return to the ED immediately if symptoms worsen.

What not to do:

- Do not lose the patient to followup. Although lower UTIs often resolve without treatment, upper UTIs inadequately treated can lead to renal damage, or sepsis.
- Do not miss an infection above a ureteral stone or obstruction. Crampy, colicky pain or hematuria with the symptoms above calls for an excretory urogram (IVP). Antibiotics and hydration alone may not cure an infected obstruction.

Discussion:

Although oral antibiotics are usually sufficient treatment for upper UTIs, there is a significant incidence of renal damage and sepsis as sequelae, mandating good followup or admission when necessary. By the same token, lower UTIs can ascend into upper UTIs, or it can be difficult to decide the level of a given UTI, in which case it should be treated as an upper UTI.

Colorful Urine

Presentation:

The patient may complain about the color of his urine; color may be one component of some urinary complaint; or the color may be noted incidentally on urinalysis.

What to do:

- Ask about symptoms of urinary urgency, frequency, and crampy pains (suggesting stones), as well as any food colorings, over-the-counter or prescription medications, or diagnostic dyes recently ingested. Ascertain the circumstances surrounding noticing the color—did the color only appear after the urine contacted the container, or the water in the toilet bowl? Did the urine have to sit in the sun for hours before the color appeared?
- Obtain a fresh urine sample for analysis. Persistent foam suggests protein or bilirubin, which should also show up on a dipstick test. A positive dipstick for blood implies the presence of red cells, free hemoglobin, or myoglobin, which can be double-checked by examining the urinary sediment for red cells and the serum for hemoglobinemia.
- If the urine is red and alkaline but does not contain hemoglobin myoglobin, or red blood cells, suspect an indicator dye such as phenolphthalein (the laxative in ExLax) in which case the red should disappear when the urine is acidified. People with a particular metabolic defect produce red urine whenever they eat beets.
- Orange urine may be produced by phenazopyridine (Pyridium) or ethoxazene (Serenium), both of which are used as urinary tract anesthetics to diminish dysuria. Rifampin will also turn urine orange.
- Blue or green urine may be caused by a blue dye such as methylene blue, a component in several medications (e.g., Trac Tabs, Urised, Uroblue) used to reduce symptoms of cystitis. A blue pigment may also be produced by Pseudomonas infection.
- Brown or black urine (not due to myoglobin or bilirubin) may be caused by L-dopa, melanin, phenacetin, or phenol poisoning. Metabolites of Aldomet may turn black on contact with bleach (which is often in toilet bowls).

What not to do:

- If suspicious, do not allow the patient to alter his urine factitiously. Have someone observe urine collection and inspect the specimen at once.

- Do not let the dipstick sit too long in the urine (allowing chemical indicators to diffuse out) or hold the dipstick vertically (allowing chemicals to drip from one pad to another and interfere with reagents).
- Do not be misled by dye in urine interfering with dipstick indicators. Pyridium can make a dipstick appear falsely positive for bilirubin, while contamination with hypochlorite bleach can cause a false positive test for hemoglobin. Also the urobilinogen dipstick (or Erlich reaction) is not adequate for diagnosing porphyria.

Urethritis (Drip)

Presentation:

A male complains of dysuria, a burning discomfort along the urethra, or a urethral discharge. A copious, thick, yellow-green discharge which stains underwear is characteristic of gonorrhea, whereas a thin, white, scant discharge with milder symptoms is characteristic of chlamydia.

Urethritis in a female may be indistinguishable from cystitis or vaginitis, but may be manifest as UTI symptoms with a low concentration of bacteria on urine culture, or tenderness localized to the anterior vaginal wall.

What to do:

- Gram stain any urethral discharge, looking for gram-negative diplococci inside white cells, which imply gonococcal infection, best treated with procaine penicillin 4.8Mu im, amoxicillin 3gm po, or ampicillin 3.5gm po (all preceded by 1gm of probenecid po), or with spectinomycin 2gm im, or tetracycline 500mg qid x 7d.
- Do a VDRL to look for established syphilis. All the above regimens (except spectinomycin) will eradicate incubating syphilis, but further antibiotic treatment is required if the VDRL is positive.
- Examine the urine sediment for swimming protozoa, implying infection with *Trichomonas vaginalis*, best treated with metronidazole (Flagyl) 250mg qid x 7d, or 2gm po once.
- Culture the discharge or swab the urethra with a small

nasopharyngeal swab, plated on Thayer-Martin media and quickly transfer to a warm CO_2-rich incubator, to establish the diagnosis or find unsuspected gonorrhea.

- If there is no sign of gonorrhea or trichomonas causing the urethritis, assume the infection is caused by chlamydia or ureaplasm, best treated with tetracycline 500mg qid x 10d.
- Ask about sexual partners who should also be treated.

What not to do:

- Do not send off a VDRL without following up on the results.

Discussion:

Our understanding of "nonspecific" urethritis (NSU) is advancing, as it becomes the most common form of urethritis in many populations. Culturing for chlamydia remains expensive, and presumptive treatment with tetracycline remains the best strategy. Many gonorrhea victims develop a rebound urethritis, probably with chlamydia, following penicillin, amoxicillin, ampicillin, or spectinomycin treatment. Thus, when the etiology of urethritis is unclear, a week to 10 days of tetracycline is probably the best empirical treatment.

Gonorrhea (Clap)

Presentation:

A young man may present with symptoms of urethritis (dysuria, discharge), or perhaps prostatitis (low back pain) or epididymitis (scrotal pain). A young woman may have cervicitis or pelvic infection (low abdominal pain, dysuria, discharge). Both sexes may present with gonococcal proctitis (rectal pain, rectal discharge, tenesmus) or pharyngitis.

What to do:

- Obtain a sexual history and look for rash, arthritis, tenosynovitis, perihepatitis, or pain on moving the cervix, which are signs of disseminated or pelvic infection, requiring a longer course of treatment or hospital admission.
- Gram stain any discharge or exudate and examine for many

gram-negative diplococci ingested by polymorphonuclear leukocytes, which corroborate the diagnosis of gonorrhea (their absence does not rule out the possibility).

- Culture the throat, urethra, cervix, anus—wherever the patient is symptomatic or exposed, according to the history. To avoid killing the organism, use a special transport medium or plate immediately on room-temperature Thayer-Martin medium which will be incubated soon.
- With female patients send a urine test to rule out pregnancy (see below).
- Send blood for syphilis serology (e.g., VDRL) and be sure someone will review and act upon the results. [Incubating syphilis (i.e., with negative VDRL) will be eradicated by all the regimens listed here (except spectinomycin) but established syphilis (i.e., with positive VDRL) will require a longer course of antibiotics.]
- Treat gonorrhea with 4.8 million units of procaine penicillin im (half in each buttock) and 1gm of probenecid po.
- Alternate regimens for patients who wish to avoid shots (but not effective for pharyngeal or anorectal gonorrhea) are ampicillin 3.5gm po or amoxicillin 3gm po, each with the same 1gm of probenecid.
- Alternate regimens for penicillin-allergic patients or penicillin-resistant gonococcus are spectinomycin 2gm im or cefoxitin 2gm im.
- For urethritis or pelvic infection where chlamydia is a likely pathogen, cover both possibilities with tetracycline 500mg qid for 10 days (but avoid tetracycline during pregnancy).
- Instruct the patient to avoid sexual contact for five days, arrange for a followup re-examination and re-culture to ensure eradication, and report the infection, if required by law.
- Treat sexual partners of patients exposed to gonorrhea with the same antibiotic regimens (you may omit cultures).

What not to do:

- Do not pretend to rule out venereal disease on the basis of a "negative" sexual history. Simply taking cultures during the physical examination is often preferable to badgering patients about intimate details they would rather not reveal.
- Do not be misled by extracellular gram-negative diplococci, which can be among the normal flora of the pharynx or vagina.
- Do not send culture or VDRL tests unless someone will see and act on the results.

Discussion:

Gonorrhea with pharyngeal or rectal involvement still responds best to probenecid and penicillin. Gonorrhea with arthritis and dermatitis requires a week of antibiotic therapy. As gonorrhea becomes more resistant to penicillin and other antibiotics, cefoxitin remains a good backup antibiotic.

Genital Herpes Simplex

Presentation:

The patient may be concerned about paresthesias and subtle genital lesions, desirous of pain relief during a recurrence, or suffering complications such as superinfection or urinary retention.

Instead of the classic grouped vesicles on an erythematous base, herpes in the genitals usually appears as groupings of 2–3mm ulcers, representing the bases of abraded vesicles. Resolving lesions are also less likely to crust on the genitals. Lesions can be tender, and should be examined with gloves on, because they shed infectious viral particles.

What to do:

- If necessary for the diagnosis, perform a Tzanck prep, by scraping the base of the vesicle (this hurts!), spreading the cells on a slide, drying, and staining with Wright's or Giemsa stain. The presence of multinucleate giant cells with nuclear molding (see p 91) confirms the diagnosis of herpes.
- Alternatively, use this sample for herpes virus culture, if available. This is becoming as rapid and inexpensive as bacterial culture in many labs. The medium is stored frozen, thawed, inoculated, and kept cold until it reaches the lab.
- Send a VDRL and culture the cervix or any urethral discharge in search of other infections requiring different therapy.
- For a first episode of herpes simplex genitalis, prescribe acyclovir (Zovirax) 5% ointment to cover all lesions q3h (6 times daily) for 7 days.
- Prescribe antiinflammatory analgesics (aspirin to Percodan) for pain.
- Warn the patient that:

a) lesions and pain can be expected to last 2 weeks during the initial attack (usually less in recurrences);
b) although acyclovir reduces shedding, he should assume he is contagious whenever there are open lesions (and can potentially transmit the virus other times as well);
c) he should be careful about touching lesions and washing hands, because other skin can be inoculated; and
d) recurrences can be triggered by any sort of local or systemic stress, and will not be helped by topical acyclovir.

- Arrange for followup. Local and national self-help groups can be useful.

What not to do:

- Do not panic the patient with a presumptive diagnosis. Take Tzanck preps and cultures first. If they confirm the diagnosis, don't make the patient feel like an outcast.
- Do not make the lesions worse with folk remedies (e.g., ether, photoinactivation, etc.).

Discussion:

Genital herpes has recently become a media event and something of a sexual "leprosy," with enormous emotional overlay, which must be taken into account when counseling patients. For example, patients with recurrences may demand acyclovir, and benefit from its placebo effect.

Acyclovir is activated by phosphorylation inside infected cells and acts by blocking viral DNA replication, but it is ineffective once viral latency is established. Latent herpes virus DNA already residing in the sensory ganglia can cause recurrences with impunity, and topical acyclovir only decreases the amount of viral shedding.

Epididymitis

Presentation:

An adult male complains of dull to severe scrotal pain developing over a period of hours to a day, and radiating to the ipsilateral lower abdomen or flank. There may be a history of recent urethritis, prostatitis or prostatectomy (allowing ingress to bacteria) or straining with lifting a heavy object, or sexual activity with a full bladder (allowing reflux of urine). There may be fever, nausea, or urinary urgency or frequency.

The epididymis, is tender, swollen, warm, and difficult to separate from the firm, nontender testicle. Increasing inflammation can extend up the spermatic cord and fill the entire scrotum, making examinations more difficult, as well as produce frank prostatitis or cystitis. The rectal exam therefore may reveal a very tender, boggy prostate.

What to do:

- Ascertain that the testicle is normal in position and perfusion. Doppler ultrasound may help pick up a drop-off in arterial flow from spermatic cord to testicle in testicular torsion.
- Palpate and ausculate, the scrotum to rule out a hernia. Gently palpate the prostate once. Culture urine and/or any urethral discharge to identify a bacterial organism.
- On rare occasions, for severe pain, you may infiltrate the spermatic cord above the inflammation with local anesthetic for better palpation and diagnosis (e.g., 1% lidocaine without epinephrine). Lesser pain may respond to antiinflammatory analgesics (e.g., Motrin, aspirin with codeine).
- Prescribe antibiotics for likely organisms. In men under 35, tetracycline 500mg qid for 10 days should eradicate N. gonorrhea and C. trachomatis. In men over 35, trimethoprim 160mg/ sulfamethoxazole 800mg bid x 10d may be better for gram-negative bacteria.
- Arrange for 2–3 days of strict bedrest, with the scrotum elevated, and urologic followup.

What not to do:

- Do not miss testicular torsion. It is far better to have the urologist explore the scrotum and find epididymitis than to delay and lose a testicle to ischemia (which can happen in only 4 hours).

Discussion:

Testicular torsion is more likely in children and adolescents, and has a more sudden onset, although it can be recurrent and is often related to exertion. If the spermatic cord is twisted, the testicle may be high, and the epididymis may be in other than its normal posterior position. A testicular scan can help differentiate torsion from the sometimes similar presentation of acute epididymitis. When torsion is suspected you may try a therapeutic detorsion by externally rotating the testicle 180 degrees with the patient standing.

Prostatitis

Presentation:

A man complains of fever, chills, perineal or low back pain, and may have urinary urgency and frequency, as well as signs of obstruction to urinary flow ranging from a weak stream to urinary retention. On gentle examination, the prostate is swollen and tender. The infection may spread from or into, the contiguous urogenital tract (epididymis, bladder, urethra), or the bloodstream.

What to do:

- Perform a rectal examination and only once, gently palpate the prostate.
- Culture the urine to help identify the organism responsible (although there is no guarantee that the bacteria in the prostate will be in the urine).
- Begin empirical treatment with trimethoprim 160mg/sulfamethoxazole 800mg (Bactrim DS or Septra DS) bid x 10d.
- Arrange for urological followup.

What not to do:

- Do not massage, or repeatedly palpate the prostate. Rough treatment is unlikely to help drain the infection or produce the responsible organism in the urine, but is likely to extend or worsen a bacterial prostatitis, or precipitate bacteremia or septic shock.

Discussion:

Not only is it difficult to obtain the organism responsible for prostatitis; it is difficult to identify an antibiotic with the correct spectrum which will also enter the prostate. Trimethoprim/sulfamethoxazole is the current favorite, but minocycline, doxycycline, and rifampin are also popular alternatives.

Blood in the ejaculate may be a sign of inflammation in the prostate and epididymis or, especially in younger males, may simply be a self-limiting sequela of vigorous sexual activity.

Urinary Retention

Presentation:

The patient may complain of increasing dull low abdominal discomfort and the urge to urinate, without having been able to urinate for many hours. A firm, distended bladder can be palpated between the symphysis pubis and umbilicus. Rectal exam may reveal an enlarged and/or tender prostate or suspected tumor.

What to do:

- Delaying only long enough for good aseptic technique, pass a Foley catheter into the bladder and collect the urine in a closed bag.
- If passage is difficult in a male patient, distend the urethra with lubricant (K-Y jelly or diluted lidocaine jelly) in a catheter-tipped syringe and try a 16, 18, or 20 French Foley.

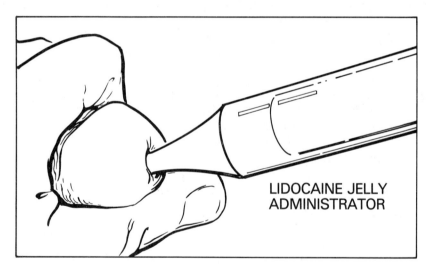

LIDOCAINE JELLY
ADMINISTRATOR

- If the problem is negotiating the curve around a large prostate, use a Coudé catheter.
- If you still cannot drain the bladder, obtain urologic consultation for stylets, sounds, filiforms, and followers.
- If the bladder drainage is voluminous, or becomes bloody, consider briefly clamping the Foley catheter every half-liter or so, to reduce the rate of fluid shifts and bladder contraction. Complications or a long period of decompression and observation may require hospitalization.

- Check renal and urinary function with a urine culture and serum BUN and creatinine determinations. Examine the patient to ascertain the cause of obstruction.
- If the volume drained is modest (1–2) and the patient stable and ambulatory, attach the Foley catheter to a leg bag and discharge him, for followup (and probably, catheter removal) the next day.
- If the volume drained is small (100–200ml), remove the catheter and search for alternate etiologies of the abdominal mass and urinary urgency.

What not to do:

- Do not use stylets or sounds unless you have experience instrumenting the urethra—these devices can cause considerable trauma.
- Do not remove the catheter in the ED if the bladder was significantly distended. Bladder tone will take several hours to return, and the bladder may become distended again.
- Do not use bethanechol (Urecholine) unless it is clear that there is no obstruction, the only cause of the distension is inadequate (parasympathetic) bladder tone and there is no possibility of gastrointestinal disease.
- Do not routinely treat the bacteria cultured from a distended bladder—they may only represent colonization which will resolve with drainage.

Discussion:

Urinary retention may be caused by stones lodged in the urethra or urethral strictures (often from gonorrhea); prostatitis, prostatic carcinoma, or benign prostatic hypertrophy; and tumor or clot in the bladder. Any drug with anticholinergic effects or alpha adrenergic effects can precipitate urinary retention. Neurologic etiologies include cord lesions and multiple sclerosis. Women with genital herpes may develop urinary retention from both loss of bladder tone and severe dysuria. Urinary retention has also been reported following vigorous anal intercourse. The urethral catheterization outlined above is appropriate initial treatment for all these conditions.

Sometimes hematuria develops midway through bladder decompression, probably representing loss of tamponade of vessels injured as the bladder distended. This should be watched until the bleeding stops (usually spontaneously) to be sure there is no great blood loss, no other urologic pathology responsible, and no clot obstruction.

Phimosis and Paraphimosis

Presentation:

Paraphimosis occurs when the foreskin cannot be replaced in its normal position after it is retracted behind the glans. The tight ring of preputial skin which is caught behind the glans creates a venous tourniquet effect and leads to edematous swelling of the glans.

Phimosis, which is the inability to retract the foreskin over the glans, is usually due to a contracted preputial opening. Patients with phimosis may seek acute medical care when they develop signs and symptoms of infection, such as pain and swelling of the foreskin and a purulent discharge.

What to do:

- For paraphimosis, squeeze the glans firmly for at least five minutes to reduce the edematous swelling. Then push the glans proximally and slide the prepuce back over the glans. If manual reduction fails, incision of the constricting tissue is necessary.
- Treating phimosis usually involves the management of acute infection. Frequent hot compresses and/or soaks are needed along with antibiotics such as cefadroxil (Duricef) or tetracycline.
- In both paraphimosis and phimosis, followup care should be provided. When swelling and inflammation subside, circumcision should be performed.

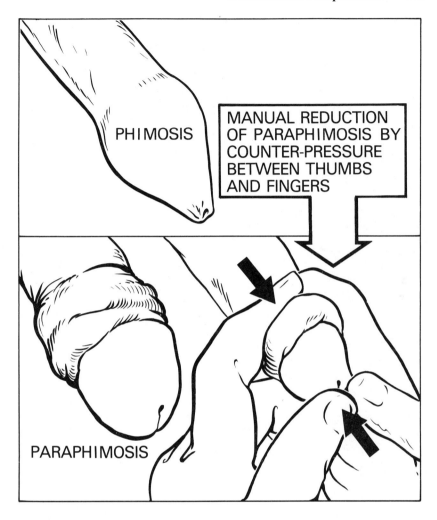

PHIMOSIS

MANUAL REDUCTION OF PARAPHIMOSIS BY COUNTER-PRESSURE BETWEEN THUMBS AND FINGERS

PARAPHIMOSIS

Discussion:

Poor hygiene and chronic inflammation are the usual causes of stenosing fibrosis of the preputial opening. In the case of a neglected paraphimosis, arterial occlusion may supervene and gangrene of the glans may develop.

Gynecologic

Dysmenorrhea (Menstrual Cramps)

Presentation:

A young woman complains of crampy, labor-like pains during her menstrual period. The pain is focused in the lower abdomen, low back, suprapubic area or thighs, and may be associated with nausea, vomiting, increased defecation, headache, muscular cramps, and passage of clots. Often, this is a recurrent problem, usually dating back to the onset of menses.

What to do:

- Ask about the duration of symptoms and onset of similar episodes (onset of dysmenorrhea after menarche suggests other pelvic pathology). Ask about appetite, diarrhea, dysuria, dyspareunia and other symptoms suggestive of other pelvic pathology.
- Perform a thorough abdominal and speculum and bimanual pelvic examination, looking for signs of infection, pregnancy, or uterine or adnexal disease.
- Confirm that the patient is not pregnant with a urine pregnancy test (or serum beta hCG if available stat).
- For uncomplicated dysmenorrhea, try nonsteroidal anti-inflammatory medications such as indomethacin (Indocin) 50mg, naproxen (Naprosyn) 500mg, or mefanemic acid (Ponstel) 500mg initially, tapering to maintenance doses (half the loading dose q6h).
- Arrange for workup of endometriosis or other underlying causes and suggest aspirin or oral contraceptives for prophylaxis.

What not to do:

- Do not treat acute dysmenorrhea with aspirin alone. Aspirin begun three days before the period, 650mg qid, is effective prophylaxis, but it is not as good once symptoms exist.

Discussion:

Prostaglandins E and F in menstrual blood appear to stimulate uterine hyperactivity, and thus many of the symptoms of dysmenorrhea.

Vaginal Bleeding

Presentation:

A menstruating woman complains of greater than usual bleeding, which is either off her usual schedule (metrorrhagia), lasts longer than a typical period, or is heavier than usual (menorrhagia), perhaps with crampy pains and passage of clots.

What to do:

- Obtain orthostatic pulse and blood pressure measurements, a hematocrit, and pregnancy test (urine or serum beta hCG level). Try to quantify the amount of bleeding by number of saturated saturated pads used.
- If there is significant bleeding, demonstrated by tachycardia, lightheadedness, orthostatic pressure changes, a pulse increase of more than 20 per minute on standing, or a hematocrit below 30%, start an intravenous line of lactated Ringer's solution, and have blood ready to transfuse.
- Obtain a menstrual, sexual, and reproductive history. Are her periods usually irregular, occasionally this heavy? Does she take oral contraceptive pills, and has she missed enough to produce estrogen withdrawal bleeding? Is an IUD in place and contributing to cramps, bleeding, and infection? Was her last period missed or light, or this period late, suggesting an anovulatory cycle? Might she be pregnant?
- Perform a speculum and manual vaginal examination, looking particularly for signs of pregnancy, such as a soft, blue cervix, enlarged uterus, or passage of fetal parts with the blood. Ascertain that the blood is coming from the cervical os, and not from a laceration polyp, or other vaginal or uterine pathology or infection. Feel for adnexal masses, as well as pelvic fluid or tenderness.

- If there is an intrauterine pregnancy, determine whether this bleeding represents an incomplete, inevitable, or threatened abortion. Spread any questionable products of conception on gauze or suspend in saline to differentiate from organized clot. Press an 8mm curette or dilator against the cervix to see whether the internal os is open (indicating an inevitable or incomplete abortion) or closed (threatened abortion, with roughly even odds of survival, and generally treated by bed-rest).
- Confirm suspicion of ectopic pregnancy either with a sonogram showing the ectopic gestational sac, a sonogram showing an empty uterus despite a positive pregnancy test, or a culdocentesis, which cannot rule out an ectopic pregnancy, but which can quickly demonstrate blood in the cul-de-sac after an ectopic sac ruptures.
- Severe dysfunctional uterine bleeding (DUB) may be slowed with intravenous estrogen (Premarin) 25mg iv every 30 minutes, up to three doses. If this does not work, or a transfusion is required, the patient should be admitted to the hospital. The patient may be discharged home on oral contraceptive pills (e.g., Ortho-Novum 1/50 or Norinyl 1 + 50, two pills bid or one qid until the bleeding stops, and then continuing one qid for two or three menstrual cycles).
- If the cause of the uterine bleeding was missed oral contraceptive pills, the patient may resume the pills, but should use additional contraception for the first cycle. (If the cause is a new IUD, the patient may elect to have it removed and use another contraceptive.)
- The patient should be referred for followup to a gynecologist, and should be evaluated via endometrial biopsy.

What not to do:

- Do not leap to a diagnosis of DUB without ruling out pregnancy.
- Do not rule out pregnancy or venereal infection on the basis of a negative sexual history—confirm with physical examination and laboratory tests.

Discussion:

The essential steps in the emergency evaluation of vaginal bleeding are fluid resuscitation of shock, if present, and recognition of pregnancy and its complications of spontaneous abortion or ectopic pregnancy (the incidence of which is increasing). Treatment of more chronic and less severe dysfunctional uterine bleeding usually consists of iron replacement and optional use of oral contraceptives to decrease menstrual irregularity (metrorrhagia) and volume (menorrhagia).

Vaginitis

Presentation:

A woman complains of itching and irritation of the labia and vagina, perhaps with vaginal discharge, vague low abdominal discomfort, or dysuria. (Suprapubic discomfort and urinary urgency and frequency suggest cystitis.) Speculum examination discloses a diffusely red, inflamed vaginal mucosa, with vaginal mucus either copious, thin, and foul-smelling (characteristic of *Trichomonas* or *Gardnerella)* or thick, white, and cheesy (characteristic of *Candida).*

What to do:

- Perform speculum and bimanual pelvic exam. Collect urine for possible culture and pregnancy tests which may influence treatment. Swab cervix and/or urethra to culture for *N. gonorrheae.* Touch pH indicator paper to the vaginal mucus (pH>4.5 suggests "nonspecific" vaginitis).
- Dab a drop of vaginal mucus on a slide, add a drop of 0.9% saline and a cover slip, and examine under 400x for swimming protozoa *(Trichomonas vaginalis),* epithelial cells covered by adherent bacilli ("clue cells" of *Gardnerella vaginalis* infection), or pseudohyphae and spores ("spaghetti and meatballs" appearance of *Candida albicans).*
- If epithelial cells obscure the view of Candida; add a drop of 10% KOH, smell whether this liberates the odor of stale fish (characteristic of Gardnerella) and look again under the microscope.
- Gram stain a second specimen. This is an even more sensitive method for detecting Candida, and clue cells, as well as a means to assess the general vaginal flora, which is normally mixed, with occasional predominance of gram-positive rods. Many white cells and an overabundance of pleomorphic gram-negative rods suggests Gardnerella infection. Gram-negative diplococci inside white cells suggests gonorrhea.
- If *Trichomonas vaginalis* is the etiology, discuss with the patient the options of metronidazole (Flagyl) 250mg tid, or 500mg bid x 7d, or 2gm once. (The last has not quite as good a cure rate, but shortens the time she must abstain from alcohol because of metronidazole's disulfiram-like activity.) Sexual partners should receive the same treatment.

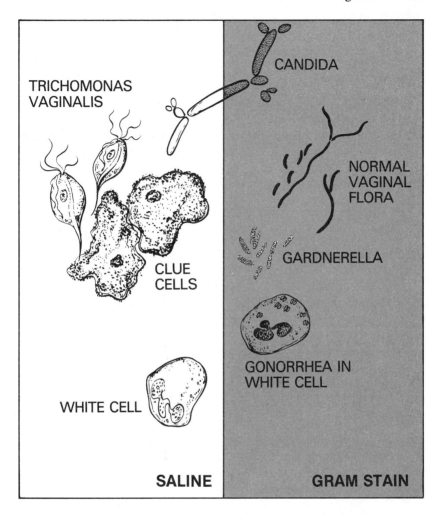

- If *Candida albicans* is the etiology, prescribe clotrimazole (Gyne-Lotrimin) or miconazole (Monistat) as 100mg vaginal tablets to be inserted qhs x 7d. Give two more tablets to use prophylactically before and after the next period.
- If overgrowth of *Gardnerella vaginalis* is present, the best treatment is metronidazole (Flagyl) 250mg tid or 500mg bid x 7–10d, although ampicillin 500mg qid and tetracycline 500mg qid are also used. With these last two regimens, it is prudent to add douching with half-strength vinegar or Betadine (one tablespoon per quart) qhs to prevent rebound *Candida* vaginitis, as the antibiotics decimate the normal vaginal flora.
- For vaginitis without evidence of any of the three organisms above, a prudent treatment is vinegar or Betadine douching alone for a week, which will help flush out possible pathogens and restore the normally acid pH of the vagina.

- Arrange for followup and instruct the patient in prevention of vaginitis.

What not to do:

- Do not prescribe sulfa creams for "non-specific" vaginitis. The treatments above are more effective.
- Do not miss underlying pelvic inflammatory disease, pregnancy, or diabetes, all of which can potentiate vaginitis.

Discussion:

The ecology of the vagina and etiology of what has long been called "non-specific" vaginitis are still not well understood. Both *Candida albicans* and *Gardnerella vaginalis* (previously known as *Hemophilus vaginalis* or *Corynebacterium vaginale*), which are often part of the normal vaginal flora and a number of anaerobes share the blame in vaginitis (thus the efficacy of metronidazole). An alternate therapy uses active-culture yogurt douches to repopulate the vagina with lactobacilli.

Vaginitis is more common in the summer, under tight or non-porous clothing (jeans, synthetic underwear, wet bathing suits), and in users of oral contraceptives (which alter vaginal mucus). Trichomonas (and possibly other etiologies) can be passed back and forth between sexual partners, a cycle that can be broken by treating both.

Vaginal Foreign Bodies

Presentation:

This commonly is a problem of children, who may insert a foreign body and not tell their parents. The patient is finally brought to the emergency department with a foul-smelling purulent discharge with or without vaginal bleeding.

Vaginal foreign bodies in the adult may be a result of a psychiatric disorder or unusual sexual practices. Occasionally a tampon or pessary is forgotten or lost and causes discomfort and a vaginal discharge.

What to do:

- Visualize the foreign body using a nasal speculum in the pediatric patient or a vaginal speculum in the adult.

- Remove the foreign body using a single clamp.
- Swab the vagina with a betadine solution.
- Consider getting x rays of the pelvis if radiopaque foreign bodies of the urethra or bladder are suspected.

What not to do:

- Do not ignore a vaginal discharge in a pediatric patient or assume it is the result of a benign vaginitis. Look for a foreign body and consider the possibility of child abuse.

Discussion:

Vaginal foreign body removal is generally not a problem, but when large objects make removal more difficult, use the additional techniques described on p 130.

Bartholin Abscess

Presentation:

A woman complains of vulvar pain and swelling that has developed over the past 2–3 days, making walking and sitting very uncomfortable.

On physical exam in the lithotomy position, there is a unilateral (occasionally bilateral), tender, fluctuant, erythematous swelling at 5 or 7 o'clock within the posterior labium minus.

What to do:

- If the swelling is mild without fluctuance (bartholinitis) or if the abscess is not pointing, the patient can be placed on an antibiotic (e.g., amoxicillin) and instructed to take warm sitz baths. Early followup should be provided.
- When the abscess is pointing, an incision should be made over the medial bulging surface and the pus evacuated.
- After drainage a Word catheter should be inserted through the incision. Inflate the tip of the catheter with sterile water to hold it in place and prevent premature closure of the opening.
- Even after drainage, the patient should be placed on amoxicillin and instructed to take sitz baths. When gonorrhea is suspected, drug dosages should be adjusted accordingly and probenecid added to the regimen.
- Provide for a followup exam within 48 hours.

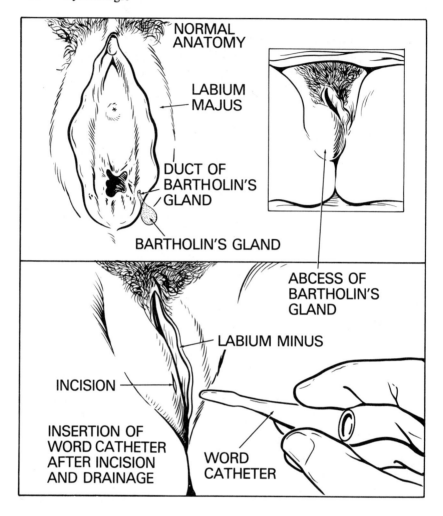

NORMAL ANATOMY

LABIUM MAJUS

DUCT OF BARTHOLIN'S GLAND

BARTHOLIN'S GLAND

ABCESS OF BARTHOLIN'S GLAND

LABIUM MINUS

INCISION

INSERTION OF WORD CATHETER AFTER INCISION AND DRAINAGE

WORD CATHETER

What not to do:

- Do not mistake a nontender Bartholin duct cyst, which does not require immediate treatment, for an inflamed abscess.
- Do not mistake a more posterior perirectal abscess for a Bartholin abscess. The perirectal abscess requires a different treatment approach.

Discussion:

The most common organisms involved in the development of a Bartholin abscess are gonococci, streptococci, and *Escherichia coli*. Bilateral infections are more commonly characteristic of gonorrhea.

Iodoform gauze can be inserted into the incised abscess as a substitute for the Word catheter. The Word catheter is left in place 4–6 weeks to help insure the development of a wide opening for continued drainage. If a wide opening persists, recurrent infections are not likely to occur, but they are common if the stoma closes.

9

Musculoskeletal

Cervical Strain (Whiplash)

Presentation:

The patient may arrive directly from a car accident, arrive the following day (complaining of increased stiffness and pain), or long after (to have injuries documented). The injury was any sort in which the neck was subjected to sudden extension and flexion, injuring intervertebral joints, discs, and ligaments, cervical muscles, or even nerve roots. As with other strains and sprains, the stiffness and pain may tend to peak on the day following the injury.

What to do:

- Obtain a detailed history to determine the mechanism and severity of the injury. Was the patient wearing a seat belt? Was the headrest up? Were eyeglasses thrown into the rear seat? Was the seat broken? Was the car damaged? Driveable afterwards? Windshield shattered?
- If there is any question at all of an unstable neck injury, start the evaluation with a crosstable film of the cervical spine. If necessary, the AP and open mouth views of the odontoid can also be obtained before the patient is moved.
- Examine the patient for involuntary splinting, point tenderness over the spinous processes, cervical muscle spasm, and/or tenderness and (to evaluate the cervical nerve roots) for strength, sensation, and reflexes in the arms.
- To evaluate the possibility of head trauma, ask about loss of consciousness and/or amnesia, and check the patient's orientation, cranial nerves, and strength and sensation in the legs as well.
- Unless the patient has reservations, or is pregnant, obtain 3 x ray views of the cervical spine: AP, lateral, and open mouth odontoid. If there is clinical nerve root impairment, or you need to see more detail of the posterior elements of the vertebrae,

obliques may also be useful. Flexion and extension views, if necessary, should only be done under careful supervision.

- If all the above is consistent with stable joint/ligament/muscle injury, explain to the patient that the stiffness and pain are often worse after 24 hours, but usually resolve over the next 3–5 days.
- Treat with immobilization (a soft cervical collar), topical ice for the first day, then heat for the later spasm, and anti-inflammatory analgesics (e.g., aspirin, Motrin).
- Arrange orthopedic followup as necessary.

What not to do:

- Do not forget to tell the patient his symptoms may well be worse a day after the injury.
- Do not skimp recording the history and physical. This sort of injury may end up in litigation, and a detailed record can obviate your being subpoenaed to testify in person.

Discussion:

X ray results for whiplash neck injuries seldom add anything to the clinical assessment but, although the frequency of radiological investigation of other minor trauma (e.g., skull films) has been decreased in some institutions, the sequelae of unrecognized cervical spine injuries are so severe that little effort has been made to reduce the use of x rays for relatively mild injuries. It is useful to discuss the pros and cons of x rays with the patient, who may prefer to do without, or may be in the ED purely to obtain radiological documentation of his injuries.

The term "whiplash" is probably best reserved for describing the mechanism of injury, and is of little value as a diagnosis. Because of the many undesirable connotations which surround this term it may be advisable not to use this term at all when writing in the medical record.

Torticollis (Wry Neck)

Presentation:

The patient complains of neck pain and is unable to turn his head, usually holding it twisted to one side, with some spasm of the neck muscles, all of which may have developed gradually, after minor turning of the head, after vigorous movement or injury, or during sleep. The pain may be in the neck muscles or down the spine, from the occiput to between the scapulae. Spasm in the occipitalis, sternocleidomastoid, trapezius, splenius cervicis, or levator scapulae muscles can be the primary cause of the torticollis; or be secondary to a slipped facette, herniated disc, or infection.

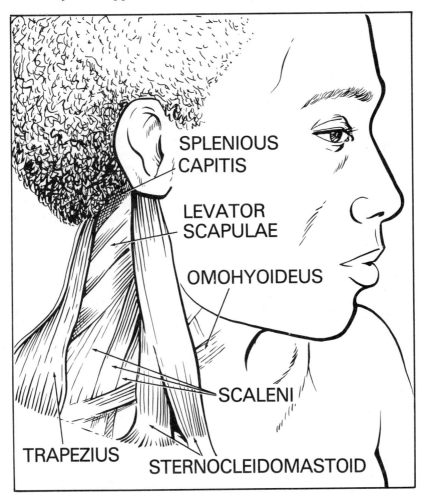

SPLENIOUS CAPITIS

LEVATOR SCAPULAE

OMOHYOIDEUS

SCALENI

TRAPEZIUS   STERNOCLEIDOMASTOID

What to do:

- Ask the patient about precipitating factors, and perform a thorough physical examination, looking for muscle spasm, point tenderness, and signs of injury, nerve root compression, or infection.

- If muscle spasm is present, apply heat (e.g., a Hydrocollator pack wrapped in several thicknesses of towel); give anti-inflammatory analgesics (e.g., aspirin, Motrin), and perhaps diazepam.
- If the onset was gradual, muscle tenderness and spasm are pronounced, neck motion seems constrained only by muscle stretching, and the symptoms are most severe when certain muscles are stretched, myalgias are probably the cause, and the routine above constitutes the treatment.
- If there is any arm weakness or paresthesia corresponding to a cervical dermatome, suspect nerve root compression as the underlying cause, and arrange for x rays and neurosurgical or orthopedic consultation.
- If there is point tenderness posterior to the sternocleidomastoid muscle (over the vertebral facets) and the head cannot turn toward the side of the point tenderness, suspect a facet syndrome, obtain x rays, and gently test neck motion again after a few minutes of manual traction (sometimes this provides some relief).
- In any event, discharge the patient with a soft cervical collar for further relief, and arrangements for x rays and followup if the torticollis has not fully resolved in 1 or 2 days.

What not to do:

- Do not overlook infectious etiologies, especially the pharyngiotonsillitis of young children, which can soften the atlanto-axial ligaments and allow subluxation, presenting as torticollis.
- Do not undertake violent spinal manipulations in the ED, which can make an acute torticollis worse.
- Do not confuse torticollis with a dystonic drug reaction (see p 12).

Discussion:

Although torticollis may signal some underlying pathology, usually it is a local musculoskeletal problem—only more frightening and noticeable for being in the neck—and need not always be totally worked up when it first presents in the ED.

Acute Lumbar Strain (Low Back Pain, Facet Syndrome)

Presentation:

Suddenly or gradually after lifting, sneezing, bending, or other movement the patient develops a dull, steady pain in the lower back. At times, this pain can be severe and incapacitating. It is usually better on lying down, worse with movement, and will perhaps radiate around the abdomen or down the thigh, but no farther. There is insufficient trauma to suspect bony injury (e.g., a fall or direct blow); and no evidence of systemic disease which would make bony pathology likely (e.g., osteoporosis, metastatic carcinoma).

On physical examination, there may be spasm (i.e., contraction which does not relax, even when the patient is supine or when the opposing muscle groups contract, as with walking in place) in the paraspinous muscles; but there is no point tenderness over the spinous processes of lumbar vertebrae and no nerve root signs [e.g., pain or paresthesia in dermatomes below the knee (especially with straight leg raising), foot weakness, or loss of the ankle jerk.]

What to do:

- Perform a complete history and physical examination of the abdomen, back, and legs, looking for alternative causes for the back pain.
- If there is point tenderness over a spinous process, neurological signs, sufficient trauma for bony injury, or any suspicion of bony pathology, obtain x rays of the lumbar spine. An AP and lateral view centered upon L3 should be sufficient.
- If the problem is injured muscles or joints, a stable compression fracture, or a herniated disc without paralysis or incontinence, start treatment with 3–5 days of *strict* bedrest, allowing only a few minutes up per day to go to the bathroom. The best position is with head flat and knees elevated on a pillow; on the side is okay, but the prone position is not good for resting the back.
- If the patient cannot accomplish strict bedrest at home, consider arranging for hospitalization or a visiting nurse.
- Prescribe anti-inflammatory analgesics (aspirin, ibuprofen) and ice to the injured area, 20 minutes per hour for the first day. (This latter therapy is unconventional, but works as well as it does for any other musculoskeletal injury.)
- Arrange for followup in 3–5 days, after the trial of bedrest.

What not to do:

- Do not be eager to use narcotic pain medicines. If the patient complies with bed rest, they are apt to make him constipated, thus especially uncomfortable with a back injury. Worse yet, they may relieve his pain, allowing him to get up and about too soon, aggravating his back problem.

- Do not be too eager to use anti-spasm medicines. Many have sedative or anticholinergic side effects, and the caveat about too-early relief of symptoms also applies.
- Do not invest too much effort in demonstrating proper lifting techniques, Williams' back exercises, etc., to the acute back strain patient in the ED. Instead, stress the proper technique of bedrest, which he needs for relief now. He should not be trying any of these activities until the acute episode has settled down.

Discussion:

Low back pain is a common and chronic problem which accounts for an enormous amount of disability and time lost from work, but the approach discussed above is geared only to the management of acute injuries and flareups.

The standard five-view x ray study of the lumbosacral spine may entail 500 mrem and exposure of gonads, and seldom produces clinically useful information except in the clinical settings of significant trauma, bony tenderness, neurological signs, or systemic disease affecting bone. Decreased disc height, compression fractures, or spondylolisthesis, for example, can all be old, non-contributory findings, depending on the clinical correlation.

History and physical examination are essential to rule out serious pathologic conditions which can present as low back pain but which require quite different treatment—aortic aneurysm, pyelonephritis, pancreatitis, pelvic inflammatory disease, ectopic pregnancy, retroperitoneal or epidural abscess.

Coccyx Fracture (Tailbone Fracture)

Presentation:

The patient fell on his tailbone and now complains of pain which is worse with sitting, and perhaps with defecation. There should be little or no pain with standing but walking may be uncomfortable. On physical examination, there is point tenderness, and perhaps deformity of the coccyx, which is best palpated by a finger in the rectum.

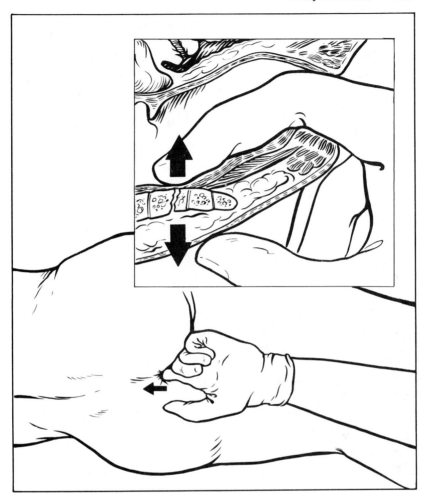

What to do:

- Verify the history (was this actually a straddle injury) and examine thoroughly, including the lumbar spine, pelvis, and the legs. Palpate the coccyx from inside and out, feeling primarily for point tenderness and/or pain on motion.
- X rays are optional. Any noticed variation can be an old fracture or an anatomic variant.
- Instruct the patient in how to sit forward, resting his weight upon ischial tuberosities and thighs, instead of on the coccyx. A foam rubber doughnut cushion may help some. If necessary, prescribe anti-inflammatory pain medications and/or stool softeners.

- Inform the patient that the pain will gradually improve over a week, as callus forms and motion decreases, and arrange for followup as needed. You may wish to inform the patient that, uncommonly, chronic pain will occur and that (rarely) it may be necessary to remove the coccyx surgically.

Fibromyalgia (Trigger Points)

Presentation:

The patient, generally between 25 and 50 years old, will be troubled with the gradual onset of fibromuscular pain that at times can be immobilizing. The areas most commonly affected include the posterior muscles of the neck and scapula, the soft tissues lateral to the thoracic and lumbar spine, and the sacroiliac joints. The patient is often depressed or under emotional or physical stress. Cold weather may be one of the precipitating causes.

There should be no swelling, erythema or heat over the painful area but applying pressure over the site with an examining finger will cause the patient to wince with pain. This tender "trigger pont" is usually no larger than your finger tip and when pressed will cause local pain, referred pain, or both.

What to do:

- When you find a trigger point, map out its exact location (point of maximum tenderness) and place an X over the site with a ball point pen. If the trigger point is diffuse there is no need to outline its location.
- Obtain a careful history and perform a general physical exam to help exclude the possibility of a serious underlying disorder such as rheumatoid arthritis or cancer.
- With any suspicion that an underlying problem exists, obtain an x ray and/or an E.S.R. These studies should both be normal in fibromyalgia.
- Where trigger points are diffuse, prescribe a nonsteroidal anti-

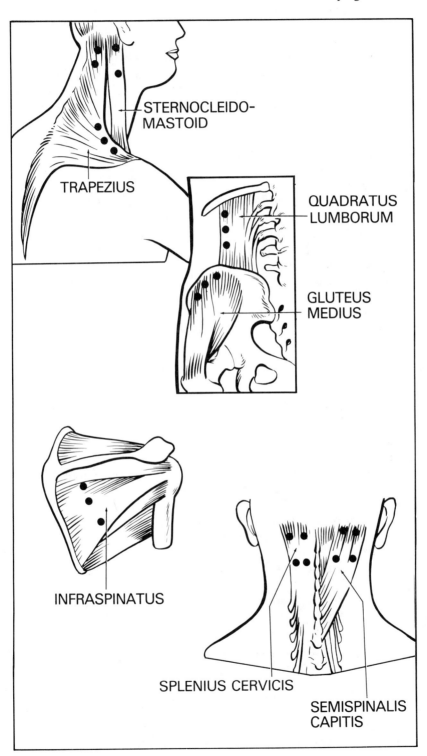

STERNOCLEIDO-
MASTOID

TRAPEZIUS

QUADRATUS
LUMBORUM

GLUTEUS
MEDIUS

INFRASPINATUS

SPLENIUS CERVICIS

SEMISPINALIS
CAPITIS

inflammatory such as naprosen 275mg (Anaprox) 2 stat, then q6h x 5 days.
- When a focal trigger point is present you can suggest to the patient that he may get immediate relief with an injection. Inject 2–4cc's of 1% xylocaine along with 40mg of methylprednisolone (Depomedrol) through the mark you placed on the skin, directly into the painful site. Be sure you are not in a vessel and then "fan" the needle in all directions while injecting the trigger point. In addition, to insure total coverage, massage the area after the injection is complete. The patient will often get complete or near-complete pain relief and a supplementary 5-day course of naprosyn (Anaprox) is optional. Complete pain relief helps to confirm the diagnosis of fibromyalgia.
- Moist hot compresses and massage may also be comforting to the patient after discharge.
- Inform the patient that after trigger point injection there may be a transient painful rebound. Anti-inflammatory analgesics will help to reduce this potential discomfort.
- Provide followup care for patients in the event their symptoms do not clear and they require further diagnostic evaluation and therapy.

What not to do:

- Do not attempt to inject a very diffuse trigger point. Results are generally unsatisfactory.

Discussion:

When the quadratus lumborum muscle is involved there is often confusion as to whether or not the patient has a renal, abdominal, or pulmonary ailment. The reason for this is the muscle's proximity to the flank and abdomen as well as its attachment to the 12th rib, which when tender, can create pleuritic symptoms. A careful physical exam, with palpation of this muscle eliciting pain, can save this patient from a multitude of laboratory and x ray studies.

Acute Monarticular Arthritis

Presentation:

The patient complains of one joint which has become acutely red, swollen, hot, painful, and stiff.

What to do:

- Ask about previous, similar episodes in this or other joints, as well as trauma, infections, or rashes, and perform a thorough physical examination looking for evidence of the same.
- Examine the affected joint, and document the extent of effusion, involvement of adjacent structures, etc.
- Cleanse the skin over the most superficial area of the joint effusion with alcohol and povidone-iodine (Betadine), anesthetize the skin with 1% plain lidocaine, and aspirate as much joint fluid as possible through an 18-gauge needle, using aseptic technique throughout.
- Grossly examine the joint aspirate. Clear, light yellow fluid is characteristic of osteoarthritis or mild inflammatory or traumatic effusions. Grossly cloudy fluid is characteristic of more severe inflammation or bacterial infection. Blood in the joint is characteristic of trauma (a tear inside the synovial capsule) or bleeding from hemophilia or anticoagulants.
- One drop of joint fluid may be used for a crude string or mucin clot test. Wet the tips of two fingers with joint fluid, and repeatedly touch them together and slowly draw them apart. As this maneuver is repeated 10 or 20 times, and the joint fluid dries, normal synovial fluid will form longer and longer strings, usually to 5–10 cm in length. Inflammation inhibits this string formation.
- The essential laboratory tests on joint fluid consist of a Gram stain and culture for possible septic arthritis. (The presence of urate crystals may sometimes be detected on the wet prep or Gram stain.)
- A joint fluid leukocyte count is the next most useful test to order. A count greater than 50,000 white cells/mm^3 is characteristic of bacterial infection (especially when most are polymorphonuclear leukocytes). In osteoarthritis, there are usually fewer than 2,000 WBCs/mm^3, and inflammatory arthritis (such as gout and rheumatoid arthritis) falls in the middle range of 2,000–50,000 WBCs/mm^3.
- Obtain x rays of the affected joint to detect possible unsuspected fractures, or evidence of chronic disease, such as osteoarthritis.
- If there is any suspicion of a bacterial infection, the patient should be begun on appropriate antibiotics which will have a high concentration in the synovial fluid. (The most common, and the most devastating, organism requiring treatment is *Staphylococcus aureus*, which may be adequately treated with oral dicloxacillin 500mg q6 hours; but, since patients with this infection must be very closely followed, it is usually more

practical to use intravenous antibiotics such as oxacillin or nafcillin. Young children with *Haemophilus influenza* infections should receive intravenous ampicillin and chloramphenicol. Young adults with *Neisseria gonorrhoeae* arthritis should receive intravenous penicillin.)

- Inflammatory arthritis may be treated with non-steroidal anti-inflammatory medications, beginning with a loading dose, such as indomethacin (Indocin) 50mg or ibuprofen (Motrin) 800mg, tapered to usual maintenance doses. Phenylbutazone should not be prescribed for more than 5 days, to avoid marrow suppression. All of these drugs irritate the gastric mucosa, but not to the same extent as colchicine, which used to be the traditional therapy for gout. Intravenous colchicine, however, in a dose of 1–2mg, produces little, if any, gastric irritation, and may be the preferred treatment in acute gouty arthritis for patients with gastritis or peptic ulcer.

- When joint fluid cannot be obtained to rule out infection, it may be a good tactic to treat simultaneously for infectious and inflammatory arthritis. Alternatively, sequential therapeutic trials may settle the diagnostic question. Prescribe an antibiotic for the first day (because infection is the more urgent possibility) and add the anti-inflammatory medication on the second day if symptoms have not improved.

- Splint and elevate the affected joint and arrange for admission or followup.

What not to do:

- Do not be misled by bursitis, tenosynovitis, or myositis without joint involvement. An infected or inflamed joint will have a reactive effusion, which may be evident as fullness, fluctuance, reduced range of motion, and/or joint fluid which can be drawn off with a needle. It is usually difficult to tap a joint in the absence of a joint effusion.

- Do not depend on serum uric acid to diagnose acute gouty arthritis—it may or may not be elevated (> 8mg/ dl) at the time of an acute arthritis.

Discussion:

The real reason for tapping a joint effusion is to rule out a bacterial infection, which could destroy the joint in a matter of days. Beyond identifying an infection (with Gram stain, culture, and WBC) further diagnosis of the cause of arthritis is not particularly accurate nor necessary to decide on acute treatment. Reducing the volume of the effusion also usually alleviates pain and stiffness, but this effect is usually short-lived, and the effusion reaccumulates within hours.

Podagra (Acute Gouty Arthritis)

Presentation:

A patient with an established diagnosis of gout or hyperuricemia develops an intensely painful monarticular arthritis, often a few hours following a minor trauma. Any joint may be affected, but most common is the metatarsophalangeal joint of the great toe. The joint is red, hot, swollen, and tender to touch or movement. There is no fever, rash, or other sign of systemic illness.

What to do:

- Provide rapid pain relief with loading doses of non-steroidal anti-inflammatory medications (e.g., Indocin 50mg po q4h or Motrin 800mg po q4h), tapering, once pain is relieved, to maintenance doses for the next few days (e.g., Indocin 25mg or Motrin 400mg tid). Excruciating pain may require one dose of narcotics while the anti-inflammatory drugs take effect.
- If the patient has a problem (with peptic ulcer or gastritis) which might contraindicate use of the non-steroidal anti-inflammatory medications, try intravenous colchicine, in a dose of 1–2mg.
- Instruct the patient to elevate and rest the painful extremity, and arrange for followup. Consider the workup for a septic arthritis (see p 171) if the inflammation does not settle down within 1–2 days.

What not to do:

- Do not use oral colchicine, which has greater gastric toxicity than the non-steroidal anti-inflammatory medications, and is not exactly specific as a therapeutic agent for gout.
- Do not prescribe phenylbutazone for more than 5 days at a time, to avoid bone marrow suppression.
- Do not start maintenance non-steroidal anti-inflammatory medications for an acute inflammation. It will take a day or more to reach therapeutic levels and pain relief.
- Do not insist upon routinely confirming a diagnosis of gout in the emergency department by ordering serum uric acid levels (which are often normal during the acute attack) or tapping an exquisitely painful joint (which may be unnecessarily cruel).
- Do not, during an acute attack of gouty arthritis, attempt to reduce the serum uric acid level with probenecid, allopurinol, etc. This will not help the arthritis, and may even be counterproductive. Leave it for followup.

Bursitis

Presentation:

Following minimal trauma or repetitive motion, a nonarticular synovial sac, or bursa, protecting a tendon or prominent bone, becomes swollen, tender, and inflamed. Because there is no joint involved, there is no decreased range of motion, but, if the tendon sheath is involved, there may be some stiffness and pain with motion.

What to do:

- Obtain a detailed history of the injury or precipitating activity, document a thorough physical examination, and rule out a joint effusion (see p 178).
- Prepare the skin with alcohol and antiseptic solution and 1% lidocaine anesthetic. Puncture the swollen bursa with a #18 or #20 needle, using aseptic technique, and withdraw some fluid to drain the effusion and rule out a bacterial infection.
- Examine a Gram stain of the effusion and send a sample for leukocyte count and culture. If there is any sign of a bacterial infection, prescribe appropriate oral antibiotics. (Bacterial infections tend to be gram-positive cocci and respond well to dicloxacillin 500mg qid x 7d.)
- Bacterial infections may also respond to direct injection of antibiotics. Severe inflammatory bursitis may require injection of local anesthetics (e.g., lidocaine, or bupivacaine) and corticosteroids (e.g., methylprednisolone (Solu-Medrol) 40mg or betamethasone (Celestone Soluspan) 0.25–0.5m).
- Construct a splint and instruct the patient in rest, elevation, and ice packing. Prescribe nonsteroidal anti-inflammatory medications, and arrange for followup.

Discussion:

Common sites for bursitis include several bursae of the shoulder and knee, the olecranon bursa of the elbow, and the trochanteric bursa of the hip. Patients with septic bursitis, unlike those with septic arthritis, can often be safely discharged on oral antibiotics, because the risk of permanent damage is much less when there is no joint involvement.

Some long-acting corticosteroid preparations can produce a rebound bursitis several hours after injection, when the local anesthetic wears off, but before the corticosteroid crystals dissolve. Patients should be so informed.

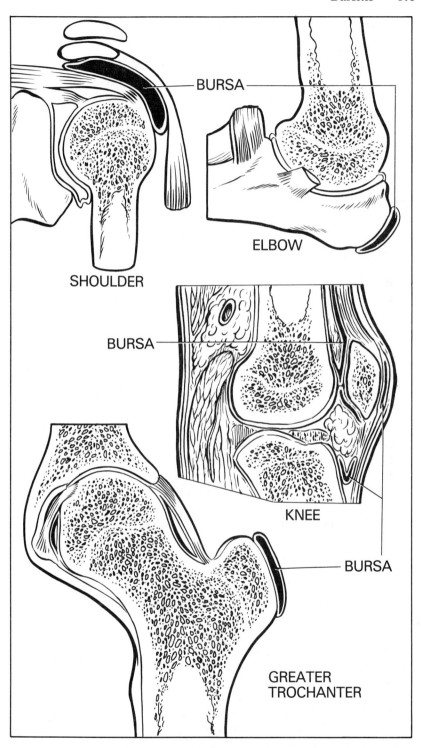

BURSA

SHOULDER

ELBOW

BURSA

KNEE

BURSA

GREATER
TROCHANTER

Ligament Sprains (Including Joint Capsule Injuries)

Presentation:

A joint is distorted beyond its normal anatomical limits (as when an ankle is inverted or a shoulder is dislocated and reduced). The patient may complain of a snapping or popping noise at the time of injury, immediate swelling, and loss of function (suggestive of a second- or third-degree sprain or a fracture); or he may come in hours to days following the injury, complaining of gradually increasing swelling and resulting pain and stiffness (suggestive of a first- or second-degree sprain and development of a traumatic effusion).

What to do:

- Obtain a detailed history of the mechanism of injury, and examine the joint for structural integrity, function, and point tenderness. Use the uninjured limb as a control.
- Obtain x rays.
- With first-degree and second-degree sprains, gently immobilize the joint using an elastic bandage alone, or in combination with a cotton roll and/or plaster splint, as discomfort demands. Shoulder injuries will require a sling, shoulder immobilizer or sling and swath. Consider prescribing anti-inflammatory pain medication when the patient complains of pain at rest and provide crutches when discomfort will not allow weight bearing.
- If there is a fracture or ligament tear with instability, the limb is usually best immobilized in a splint or cast. Splint ankles at 90 degrees and wrists in extension.
- Instruct the patient in rest, elevation, and application of ice (10–20 minutes each hour) for the first 24 hours.
- Explain to the patient that swelling in acute musculoskeletal injuries usually increases for the first 24 hours, and then decreases over the next 2–4 days (longer if the treatment above is not employed) and that some swelling and discomfort may persist for several weeks and at times for several months.
- Explain the possibility of occult injuries, the necessity for followups, and the slow healing of injured ligaments (usually 6 months until full strength is regained).

What not to do:

- Do not obtain x rays before the history or physical examination. Films of the wrong spot can be very misleading. For example, physicians have been steered away from the diagnosis of an avulsion fracture of the base of the fifth metatarsal by the presence of normal ankle films.

- Do not base the diagnosis of a ligamentous injury on x rays. They should be used as confirmatory evidence.

Discussion:

Ligamentous injuries are classified as first-degree, (minimal stretching); second-degree (a partial tear with functional loss and bleeding but still holding); and third-degree (complete tear with ligamentous instability). A tense joint effusion will limit the physical examination (and is one reason to require re-evaluation after the swelling has decreased) but also suggests less than a third-degree ligamentous injury, which is normally accompanied by a tear of the joint capsule.

Muscle Strains and Tears

Presentation:

Strains occur during or after a vigorous overstretching of a muscle bundle that leads to an insidious development of pain and tightness which is worse with use and better with rest. Tears of the muscle belly tend to be partial, with sudden onset of pain and partial loss of function. Often a tear occurs with considerable bleeding which can lead to remarkable hematomas, causing swelling at the site and dissecting along tissue planes to create ecchymoses at distant, uninvolved sites. Complete tears are more likely in the tendinous part of the muscle, and produce immediate loss of function, and retraction of the torn end, creating a deformity and bulge.

What to do:

- Obtain a history of the mechanism of injury, and test individual muscle functions. A complete tear of a muscle merits orthopedic consultation.
- Even for a partial tear of a muscle belly, try to refine the diagnosis to a specific muscle or muscle group, to help exclude other possibilities.
- For muscle strains, provide soft splinting, analgesics and instruct the patient to apply warm moist compresses for comfort.

- For muscle tears, construct a loose splint to immobilize the injured part, and instruct the patient in rest, elevation, and ice.
- Warn the patient that partial tears can become complete, and that blood will change color and percolate to the skin at distant sites, where it does not imply additional injury. Arrange for followup.

Discussion:

Some restrict the term "strain" to muscle injuries, and "sprain" to ligament injuries. A complete tear of the plantaris tendon in the leg is difficult to differentiate from a partial tear of the gastrocnemius muscle, but the treatment for both is the same.

Traumatic Effusion

Presentation:

Either immediately or one to two days after an injury such as a contusion of a bursa or the deformation of a joint, the patient complains of swelling, pain, and (in the case of a joint injury) decreased range of motion. Physical examination shows minimal or absent redness and heat, but there is a palpable or visible effusion, which may interfere with evaluation of bony or ligamentous tenderness or stability.

What to do:

- Obtain a complete history, including the mechanism of injury and subsequent treatments, and as complete a physical examination as possible.
- Obtain x rays.
- If it is necessary to rule out infection, relieve severe pain or demonstrate a complete (third-degree) ligamentous tear which will be operatively repaired in the next 2–3 days, prep the skin, tap the effusion (see p 171), examine the fluid, and/or instill 1% lidocaine and re-examine the joint for stability.
- Instruct the patient on rest, ice application for 10–20 minutes per hour the first 24–48 hours, and on the use of crutches if appropriate. Immobilize the joint with a bulky dressing or splint, and elevate the injured part until the swelling is decreased, prescribe aspirin or other anti-inflammatory medications for the pain, swelling, inflammation, and stiffness, and arrange followup in 3–4 days.

What not to do:

- Do not forget to warn patients with acute musculoskeletal injuries that stiffness, effusions, and edema typically peak at 24–48 hours. The patient who is not prepared for this may return unnecessarily, convinced he is getting worse.

Discussion:

Although a tense joint effusion interferes with testing of associated ligaments, its existence at least proves that the joint capsule is intact, and implies that the contiguous ligaments are not likely to be completely ruptured (this assurance does not apply to the knee). Tapping traumatic effusions and hemarthroses does transiently decrease pain, but the fluid usually reaccumulates within a few hours. Fat globules in the effusion indicate an occult fracture. Immediate operative repair of third-degree ligamentous tears is usually reserved for young athletes who demand as much function as possible as soon as possible. Thus the majority of joint effusions are not much helped by routine arthrocentesis.

Subluxation of the Head of the Radius (Nursemaid's Elbow)

Presentation:

A toddler will have received a sudden jerk on his arm causing enough pain that he holds it motionless. Circumstances surrounding the injury may be obvious (such as a parent pulling the child up out of a puddle); or obscure (the babysitter who reports that the child "just fell down"). The patient and family may not be accurate about localizing the injury, and complain that the child has injured his shoulder or wrist.

The patient is comfortable at rest, splinting his arm with mild flexion at the elbow and pronation of the forearm. There should be

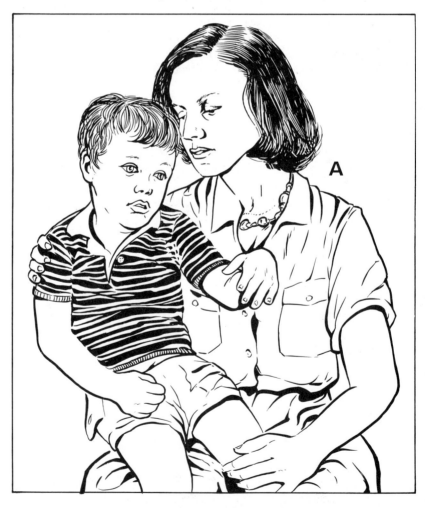

no deformity, crepitation, swelling, or discoloration of the arm. There is also no palpable tenderness except over the radiohumeral joint; the child will start to cry with any movement of the elbow joint.

What to do:

- Rule out any history of significant trauma, such as a fall from a height.
- Thoroughly examine the entire extremity, including the shoulder girdle, hand and wrist.
- If there is any suspicion of a fracture, get an x ray.
- When subluxation is suspected, place the patient in the parent's lap and inform the mother or father that it appears their child's elbow is slightly out of place and that you are going to put it back in. Warn them that this is going to hurt for a few moments.
- Put your thumb over the head of the radius and press down while you smoothly and fully extend the elbow, and at the same time supinate the forearm. Complete the procedure by fully flexing the elbow while your thumb remains pressing against the radial head and the forearm remains supinated. At some point you should feel a click beneath your thumb.

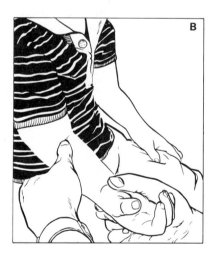
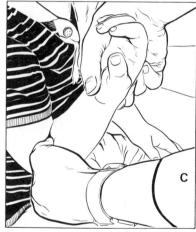

- The patient will usually scream for a while at this point. Leave for about ten minutes; then return and re-examine to see that the child has fully recovered. Post-reduction immobilization is usually unnecessary.
- Reassure the parents, explain the mechanism involved in the injury, and teach them how to prevent and treat recurrences.

- Without full recovery, get x rays.
- If x rays are negative, but the child still does not use his arm normally, place the arm in a sling and instruct the family to seek orthopedic followup care if recovery doesn't occur within 24 hours.

What not to do:

- Do not attempt to reduce an elbow where the possibility of fracture or dislocation exists.
- Do not get unnecessary x rays when all the findings are consistent with nursemaid's elbow. The x rays will appear normal, even when the radial head is indeed subluxed. Associated fractures occur, yet are not common.
- Do not confuse nursemaid's elbow with the more serious brachial plexus injury, which occurs after much greater stress and results in a flaccid paralysis of the arm.

Discussion:

This injury is an axial subluxation of the radial head away from the capitellum through the annular ligament, and occurs almost exclusively among children between 18 months and 3 years of age. On occasion, if the subluxation has been present for several hours, edema, pain, and natural splinting will continue even after reduction, or may prevent reduction.

Radial Head Fracture

Presentation:

A patient who has fallen on an outstretched hand, has a normal, non-painful shoulder, wrist, and hand, but pain in the elbow joint. The joint may be intact, with full range of flexion, but there will be pain and/or decreased range of motion on extension, supination and pronation. Tenderness, if localized, will be greatest over the radial head and lateral condyle. X rays may show a fracture or dislocation of the head of the radius. In all views, a line down the center of the radius should point to the capitellum of the lateral condyle. Often, however, no fracture is visible, and the only x ray signs are of the elbow effusion or hemarthrosis pushing the posterior fat pad out of the olecranon fossa into view; and the anterior fat pad up out of its normal alignment.

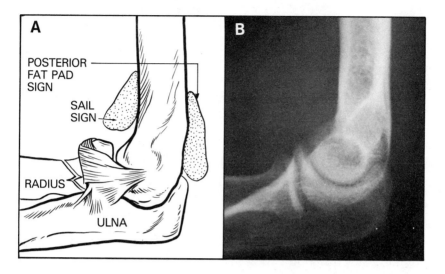

What to do:

- Obtain a detailed history of the mechanism of injury, a detailed physical examination, looking for the features described above, and x rays of the elbow, looking for visible fat pads as well as fracture lines.
- If there is any question of a radial head fracture, immobilize the elbow (including pronation and supination of the hand) with a cast, gutter splint extending from proximal humerus to hand, or sugar tong splints, for 2–3 weeks. Have the patient keep the arm in a sling for added comfort and apply ice for the first 1–2 days.

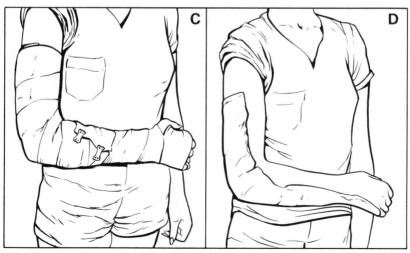

- Explain to the patient the possibility of a fracture, despite negative x rays, and arrange for followup.

What not to do:

- Do not jump to the diagnosis of "tennis elbow" or "sprained elbow" simply on the basis of a negative x ray.

Discussion:

Small, non-displaced fractures of the radial head may show up on x rays weeks later or never at all. Because pronation and supination of the hand are achieved by rotating the radial head upon the capitellum of the humerus, very small imperfections in healing of the radial head may produce enormous impairment of hand function, which may be only partly improved by surgical excision of the radial head. Immobilization at the first question of a radial head fracture may help preserve essential pronation and supination.

"Tennis elbow" is a tenosynovitis of the common insertion of the wrist extensors upon the lateral condyle, and results in pain on wrist extension rather than on pronation and supination.

Radial Neuropathy (Saturday Night Palsy)

Presentation:

The patient has injured his upper arm, usually by sleeping with his arm over the back of a chair, and now presents holding the affected hand and wrist with his good hand, complaining of decreased or absent sensation on the radial and dorsal side of his hand and wrist, and of inability to extend his wrist, thumb and finger joints. With the hand supinated (palm up) and the extensors aided by gravity, hand function may appear normal, but when the hand is pronated (palm down) the wrist and hand will drop.

What to do:

- Look for associated injuries. This sort of nerve injury may be associated with cervical spine fracture, injury to the brachial plexus in the axilla, or fracture of the humerus.
- Document in detail all motor and sensory impairment. Draw a diagram of the area of decreased sensation, and grade muscle

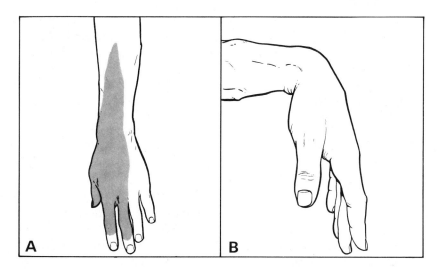

strength of various groups (flexors, extensors, etc.) on a scale of 1–5.

- If there is complete paralysis or complete anesthesia, arrange for additional neurological evaluation and treatment right away. Incomplete lesions may be satisfactorily referred for followup evaluation and physical therapy.
- Construct a splint, extending from proximal forearm to just beyond the MCP joint (leaving the thumb free) which holds the wrist in 90 degree extension. This and a sling will help protect the hand, also preventing edema and distortion of tendons, ligaments, and joint capsules which can result in loss of hand function after strength returns.

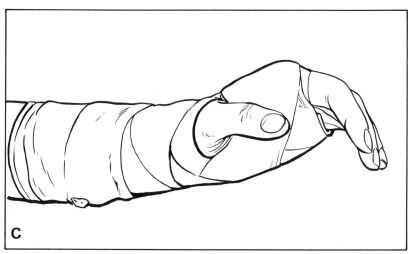

- Explain to the patient the nature of his nerve injury, the slow rate of regeneration, the importance of splinting and physical therapy for preservation of eventual function, and arrange for followup.

What not to do:

- Do not be misled by the patient's ability to extend the interphalangeal joints of the fingers, which may be accomplished by the ulnar-innervated interosseus muscles.

Discussion:

This neuropathy is produced by compression of the radial nerve as it spirals around the humerus. Most commonly it occurs when a person falls asleep, intoxicated, held up by his arm thrown over the back of a chair. Less severe forms may befall the swain who keeps his arm on his date's chair back for an entire double feature, ignoring the growing pain and paresis.

If the injury to the radial nerve is at the elbow or just below, there may be sparing of the wrist radial extensors as well as the radial nerve autonomous sensation. The deficient groups will be the wrist ulnar extensors as well as the MCP extensors. A high radial palsy in the axilla (e.g., from leaning on crutches) will involve all of the radial nerve innervations, including the triceps.

Cheiralgia Paresthetica (Handcuff Neuropathy)

Presentation:

The patient may complain of pain around the thumb while tight handcuffs were in place. The pain decreased with handcuff removal, but there is residual paresthesia or decreased sensation over the radial side of the thumb metacarpal (or a more extensive distribution). The same injury may also be produced by pulling on a loop around the wrist, or wearing a tight watchband.

What to do:

- Carefully examine and document the motor and sensory function of the hand. Draw the area of paresthesia or decreased sensation as demonstrated by light touch or two-point discrimination. Document that there is no weakness or area of complete anesthesia.

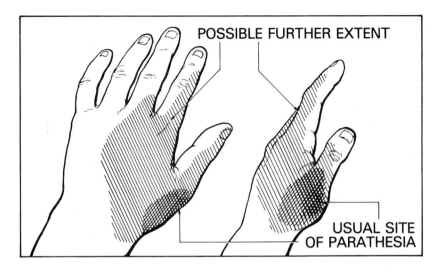

POSSIBLE FURTHER EXTENT

USUAL SITE
OF PARATHESIA

- Explain to the patient that the nerve has been bruised, that its function should return as it regenerates, but that the process is slow, requiring about two months.
- Arrange for followup if needed. Bandages, splints, or physical therapy are usually not necessary.

What not to do:

- Do not overlook more extensive injuries, such as a complete transection of the nerve (with complete anesthesia) or a more proximal radial nerve palsy (see p 184). Do not forget alternative causes, such as peripheral neuropathy, DeQuervain's tenosynovitis, carpal tunnel syndrome, scaphoid fracture, or a gamekeeper's thumb.

Discussion:

A superficial, sensory cutaneous twig of the radial nerve is the branch most easily injured by constriction of the wrist. Its area of innervation can vary widely (see figure). Axonal regeneration of contused nerves proceeds at about 1mm per day (or about an inch a month); thus recovery may require two months (measuring from site of injury in wrist to end of area of paresthesia).

Patients may want this injury documented as evidence of "police brutality," but it can be a product of their own struggling as much as too tight handcuffs.

Carpal Tunnel Syndrome

Presentation:

The patient complains of pain, tingling, or a "pins and needles" sensation in the hand. Onset may have been abrupt or gradual but the problem is most noticeable upon awakening or after extended use of the hand. The sensation may be bilateral, may include pain in the wrist, or forearm and is usually ascribed to the entire hand, until specific physical examination localizes it to the median nerve distribution. More established cases may include weakness of the thumb and atrophy of the thenar eminence.

Physical examination localizes paresthesia and decreased sensation to the median distribution (which may vary) and motor weakness, if present, to intrinsic muscles with median innervation. Innervation varies widely, but the muscles most reliably innervated by the median nerve are the abductors and opponens of the thumb.

What to do:

- Perform and document a complete examination, sketching the area of decreased sensation and grading (on a scale of 0–5) the strength of the hand.
- Hold the wrist flexed at 90 degrees for 60 seconds, to see if this reproduces symptoms. This is known as Phalen's test, and is more sensitive than the reverse (hyperextending the wrist) and more specific than tapping over the volar carpal ligament to elicit paresthesia (Tinel's Sign).
- Explain the nerve-compression etiology to the patient, and arrange for additional evaluation and followup. Borderline diagnoses may be established with electromyography (EMG), but cases with pronounced pain or weakness may require early surgical decompression. Anti-inflammatory medication, elevation of the affected hand, ice, immobilization with a volar splint, and rest may all help to reduce symptoms.

What not to do:

- Do not rule out thumb weakness just because the thumb can touch the little finger. Thumb flexors may be innervated by the ulnar nerve. Test abduction and opposition—can the thumb rise from the plane of the palm and can the thumb pad meet the little finger pad?
- Do not diagnose carpal tunnel syndrome solely on the basis of a positive Tinel's sign. Paresthesia can be produced in the distribution of any nerve if one taps hard enough.

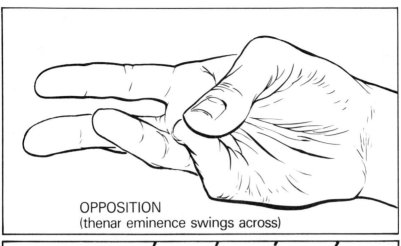

OPPOSITION
(thenar eminence swings across)

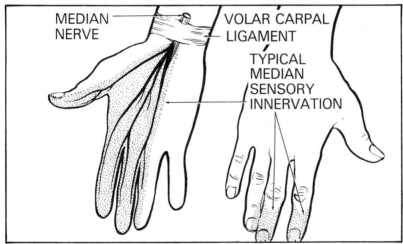

MEDIAN NERVE

VOLAR CARPAL LIGAMENT

TYPICAL MEDIAN SENSORY INNERVATION

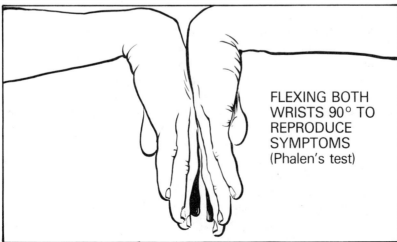

FLEXING BOTH WRISTS 90° TO REPRODUCE SYMPTOMS
(Phalen's test)

Discussion:

There is little space to spare where the median nerve and digit flexors pass beneath the volar carpal ligament, and a very little swelling may produce this specific neuropathy. Trauma, arthritis, pregnancy, and weight gain are among the many factors which can precipitate this syndrome.

Less commonly, the median nerve can be entrapped more proximally, where it enters the medial antecubital fossa through the pronator teres. Symptoms of this cubital tunnel syndrome may be reproduced with elbow extension and forearm pronation.

Ganglion Cysts

Presentation:

The patient is concerned about a rubbery, rounded swelling emerging from the general area of a tendon sheath of the wrist or hand. It may have appeared abruptly, been present for years, or fluctuated, suddenly resolving and gradually returning in pretty much the same place. There is usually little tenderness, inflammation, or interference with function, but ganglion cysts are bothersome when they get in the way and painful when repeatedly traumatized.

What to do:

- Undertake a thorough history and physical exam of the hand to ascertain that everything else is normal. X rays are of no value unless there is some question of bony pathology.
- Explain to the patient that this is a fluid-filled cyst, spontaneously arising from bursa or tendon sheath, and posing no particular danger. Treatment options include: hitting it with a large book (Harrison's *Principles of Internal Medicine* is excellent) to rupture the cyst, with a fair chance of recurrence; draining the contents of the cyst with an 18-gauge needle to reduce its size and then injecting corticosteroid, also with a good chance of recurrence; arranging for a surgical excision, which will provide definitive pathologic diagnosis, but the dissection is sometimes unexpectedly extensive, and still allows some chance of recurrence; and doing nothing, in which case the cyst may spontaneously drain and may recur.

- Follow the wishes of the patient regarding above and arrange for followup.

Discussion:

Ganglion cysts are outpouchings of bursae or tendon sheaths, with no clear etiology and no relation to nerve ganglia. Perhaps they got their name because their contents are "gluey." Reassurance about their insignificance is often the best we can offer patients.

Scaphoid (Carpal Navicular) Fracture

Presentation:

The patient (usually 14–40 years old) fell on an outstretched hand, with the wrist held rigid and extended, and now complains of pain, swelling, and decreased range of motion in the wrist, particularly on the radial side. Physical examination discloses no deformity, but pain with motion and palpation and often swelling, especially in the anatomic snuff box (on the radial side of the wrist, between the tendon of the extensor pollicis longus and the tendons of the abductor pollicis longus and extensor pollicis brevis).

What to do:

- Apply ice and a temporary splint, check for distal sensation and movement, and other injuries; and order x rays of the wrist, with special attention to the scaphoid bone and its fat pad.
- Regardless of whether a scaphoid fracture shows on x ray, splint or cast the wrist in extension, with the thumb out in opposition, and immobilized to its interphalangeal joint.
- Explain to the patient the frequent difficulty of visualizing scaphoid fractures on x rays, the frequent difficulty in healing of scaphoid fractures due to variable blood supply, and the resultant necessity of keeping this splint or cast in place for 2–3 weeks.
- Arrange for re-evaluation and further treatment within the next few days.

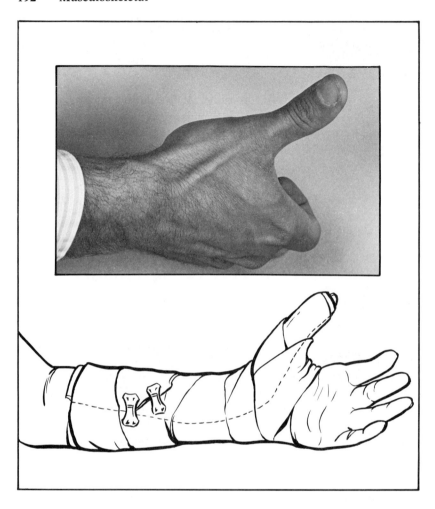

What not to do:

- Do not diagnose a "sprained wrist" on the basis of a negative x ray.
- Do not simply wrap an injured, swollen wrist. Immobilization and reduction of edema are much better if the wrist is splinted in extension and elevated as well.
- Do not assume that the thumb is adequately immobilized by a wrap or bulky dressing. Adequate immobilization of one joint above and below the scaphoid bone requires a wrist splint or cast incorporating a spica extending to the thumb interphalangeal joint.

Discussion:

Because fractures of the scaphoid bone are common; because they are often invisible on x ray until weeks later; because the blood supply to the fractured area may be tenuous and non-union or avascular necrosis likely; and because the resultant pain and arthritis may severely limit hand function; it is prudent practice to splint or cast all wrist injuries with tenderness in the anatomical snuff box with a thumb spica for at least 2–3 weeks.

Third Degree Tear of Ulnar Collateral Ligament (Skipole or Gamekeeper's Thumb)

Presentation:

The patient fell while holding onto a ski pole, banister, or other fixed object, forcing his thumb into abduction. (This same lesion may be produced by the repeated breaking of the necks of game birds—hence the name.) The metacarpophalangeal joint of the thumb is swollen, tender, and stiff; but, when tested for stability, can be deformed towards the radial (or palmar) aspect more than the MP joint of the other thumb. Having the patient pinch between the thumb and index finger, if possible at all, is less strong than with the other hand.

What to do:

- Examine thoroughly and obtain x rays, which should be negative or show a small avulsion fracture at the insertion of the ulnar collateral ligament.
- Treat with ice, elevation, rest, anti-inflammatory medications, and immobilization in a radial gutter splint, including the thumb (see figure, p 192).
- Explain to the patient that this particular injury may not heal with closed immobilization, but sometimes requires operative repair; and arrange for re-examination and orthopedic referral after a few days, when the swelling is decreased.

Discussion:

The ulnar collateral ligament of the metacarpophalangeal joint of the thumb, once completely torn, may retract its torn ends under other structures, where they are no longer apposed and cannot be depended upon to heal. An operation may be required to reappose the two ends of the ligament or reattach an avulsed insertion, but this is not usually done immediately. Left unrepaired, a gamekeeper's thumb remains unstable, and weak in pinching and holding.

For minor sprains or partial ligament tears, an elastic wrap that incorporates the thumb may be all that is required to reduce mobility and provide comfort.

Finger (PIP Joint) Dislocation

Presentation:

The patient will have jammed his finger, causing a hyperextension injury that forces the middle phalanx dorsally and proximally out of articulation with the distal end of the proximal phalanx. An obvious deformity will be seen unless the patient or a bystander has reduced the dislocation on his own. There should be no sensory or vascular compromise.

What to do:

- Unless a shaft fracture is suspected, x rays should be deferred and joint reduction should be carried out first.
- If there has been significant delay in seeking help or the patient is suffering considerable discomfort, a digital block over the proximal phalanx will allow for a more comfortable reduction.
- To reduce the joint, do not pull on the fingertip; instead, push the base of the middle phalanx distally, using your thumb until it slides smoothly into its natural anatomical position.
- Now test the finger for collateral ligament instability and avulsion of the central extensor tendon slip. The patient should be able to extend his finger at the PIP joint. Testing for avulsion of the volar carpal plate, you will be able to hyperextend the PIP joint more than that of the same finger on the uninjured hand. If any of these associated injuries exist, orthopedic consultation should be sought and prolonged splinting and rehabilitation will be required.
- Post-reduction x-rays should be taken. "Chip fractures" may represent tendon or ligament avulsions.

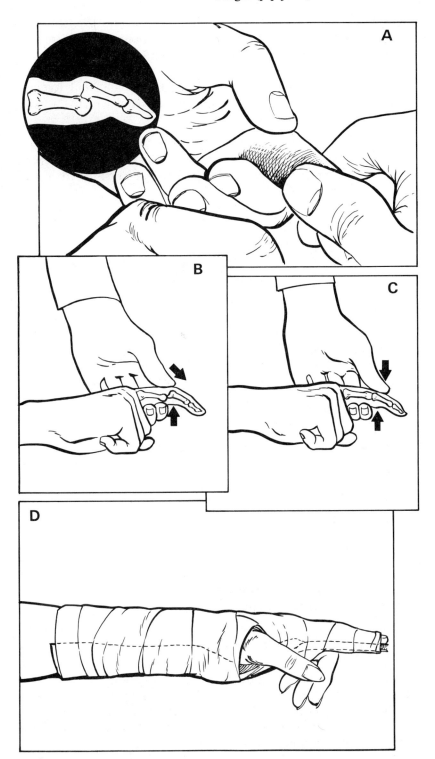

- Splint in extension for 3–4 days and provide followup for active range of motion exercises to restore normal joint mobility.
- Inform the patient that joint swelling and stiffness may persist for months after the initial injury.
- Remind the patient to keep the injured finger elevated. Recommend ice application for the next 24 hours and aspirin for pain.

Discussion:

If there is any doubt as to the competence of the central extensor slip or the volar carpal plate, the joint must be splinted in full extension for 3 weeks.

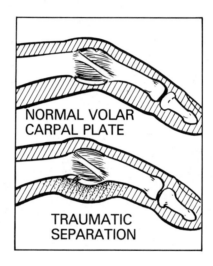

Extensor Tendon Avulsion—Distal Phalanx (Baseball or Mallet Finger)

Presentation:

There is a history of a sudden resisted flexion of the DIP joint, such as when the finger tip is jammed or struck by a ball, resulting in pain and tender ecchymotic discoloration over the dorsum of the base of the distal phalanx. When the finger is held in extension, the injured DIP joint remains in slight flexion.

What to do:

- Obtain an x ray. It may or may not demonstrate an avulsion fracture.
- Apply a finger splint that will hold the DIP joint in neutral position or slight hyperextension, and firmly tape it in place.
- Instruct the patient to keep the splint in place continuously and seek orthopedic followup care within one week.
- Prescribe an analgesic as needed.

What not to do:

- Do not assume there is no significant injury just because the x ray is negative. With or without a fracture the tendon avulsion requires splinting.
- Do not forcefully hyperextend the joint. This can result in ischemia and skin breakdown over the joint.

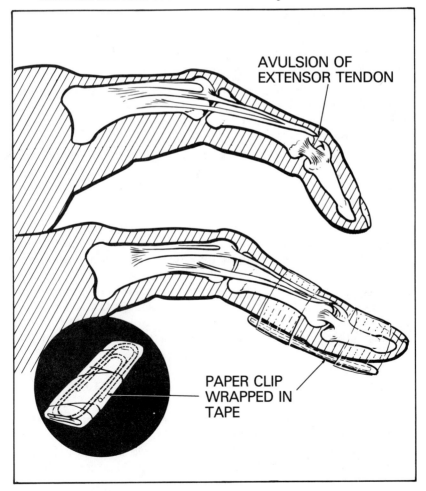

AVULSION OF
EXTENSOR TENDON

PAPER CLIP
WRAPPED IN
TAPE

Discussion:

Adequate splinting usually restores full range and strength to DIP joint extension, but the patient will require 6 weeks of immobilization, and should be informed that healing might be inadequate, requiring surgical repair.

A wide variety of splints are commercially available for splinting this injury, but, in a pinch, a tape-covered paper clip will do. A dorsal splint allows more use of the finger, but requires more padding and may contribute to ischemia of the skin overlying the DIP joint.

Plantaris Tendon Rupture

Presentation:

The patient will come in limping, having suffered a whip-like sting in his calf while stepping off hard on his foot during a game of tennis, or similar activity. He may have actually heard or felt a "snap" at the time of injury. The deep calf pain persists and may be accompanied by mild swelling and ecchymosis. Neurovascular function will be intact.

What to do:

- Rule out an Achilles tendon rupture. Test for strength in plantar flexion (can the patient walk on his toes?). Squeeze the Achilles tendon and palpate for a tender deformity that represents a torn segment. If pain does not allow active plantar flexion, squeeze the gastrocnemius muscle with the patient kneeling on a chair and look for the normal plantar flexion of the foot. This will be absent with a complete Achilles tendon tear. With any Achilles tendon tear, orthopedic consultation is necessary.
- When an Achilles tendon rupture has been ruled out, provide the patient with elastic support (e.g., ACE, TEDs stocking, Tibigrip) from foot to tibial tuberosity.
- Provide the patient with crutches for several days. Permit weight bearing only as comfort allows.
- Have the patient keep the leg elevated and at rest for the next 24–48 hours, initially applying cold packs, and after 24 hours, alternately with heat every few hours.

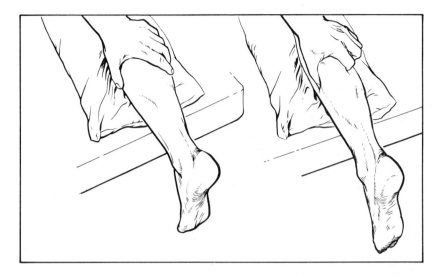

- An analgesic such as codeine may be helpful initially and heel elevation should be provided for several weeks.

What not to do:

- Do not bother getting x rays of the area unless there is a suspected associated bony injury. This is a soft tissue injury that is not generally associated with fractures.

Discussion:

The plantaris muscle is a pencil-sized structure tapering down to a fine tendon which runs beneath the gastrocnemius and soleus muscles to attach to the Achilles tendon or to the medial side of the tubercle of the calcaneus. The function of the muscle is of little importance and, with rupture of either the muscle or the tendon, the transient disability is due only to the pain of the torn fibers or swelling from the hemorrhage. Clinical differentiation from incomplete rupture of the Achilles tendon is sometimes difficult to make. Most instances of "tennis leg" are now felt to be due to partial tears of the medial belly of the gastrocnemius muscle or to ruptures of blood vessels within that muscle. The greater the initial pain and swelling, the longer one can expect the disability to last.

Broken Toe

Presentation:

The patient has stubbed, hyperflexed, hyperextended, hyperabducted, or dropped a weight upon a toe. He presents with pain, swelling, ecchymosis, decreased range of motion and point tenderness, and there may or may not be any deformity.

What to do:

- Examine the toe, particularly for lacerations which could become infected, prolonged capillary filling time in the injured or other toes which could indicate poor circulation, or decreased sensation in the injured or other toes which could indicate peripheral neuropathy, and may interfere with healing.
- X rays are not essential but are usually necessary to provide patient satisfaction. They have little effect on the initial treatment, but may help predict the duration of pain and disability (e.g., fractures entering the joint space).
- Displaced or angulated phalangeal fractures must be reduced with linear traction after a digital block. Angulation can be further corrected by using your finger as a fulcrum to reverse the direction of the distal fragment. The broken toe should fall into its normal position when it is released after reduction.
- Splint the broken toe by taping it to an adjacent non-affected toe, padding between toes with gauze or Webril, and using ½" tape. Give the patient additional padding and tape, so he may revise the splinting, and (if there is a fracture) advise him that he will require such immobilization for approximately one-two weeks, by which time there should be good callus formation around the fracture and less pain with motion. Inform the patient that he must keep the padding dry between his toes while they are taped together or the skin will become macerated and will break down.
- Also treat with rest, ice, elevation, and anti-inflammatory medication. A cane, crutches, or hard-soled shoes which minimize toe flexion may all provide comfort. Let the patient know that in many cases a soft slipper or an old sneaker with the toe cut out may be more comfortable.
- Arrange for followup if the toe is not much better within 3 weeks.

What not to do:

- Do not tape toes together without padding between them. Friction and wetness will macerate the skin between.
- Do not let the patient overdo ice, which should not be applied directly to skin, and should not be used for more than 10–20 minutes per hour.
- Do not overlook the possibility of acute gouty arthritis, which sometimes follows minor trauma after a delay of a few hours.

Discussion:

If there is no toe fracture, the treatment is the same, but the pain, swelling, and ability to walk may improve in 3–4 days rather than 1–2 weeks. A non-displaced metatarsal fracture is best treated with a splint to the foot (e.g., posterior slab or bulky soft dressing) and, if displaced, usually merits orthopedic consultation.

10

Soft Tissue

Superficial Finger Tip Avulsion

Presentation:

The mechanisms of injury can be a knife, a meat slicer, a closing door, or a falling manhole cover, or spinning fan blades, or turning gears. Depending on the angle of the amputation, varying degrees of tissue loss will occur from the volar pad, or finger tip.

What to do:

- X ray any crush injury or an injury caused by a high speed mechanical instrument, such as an electric hedge trimmer.
- Consider tetanus prophylaxis.
- Perform a digital block to obtain complete anesthesia (See p 283).
- Thoroughly debride and irrigate the wound.
- On a less than 1cm² full-thickness tissue loss, apply a simple non-adherent dressing with some gentle compression. (See p 284).
- Where there is greater than 1cm² of full-thickness skin loss there are three options that may be followed:
  a) Simply apply the same non-adherent dressing used for a smaller wound.
  b) If the avulsed piece of tissue is available and it is not severely crushed or contaminated, you can convert it into a modified full-thickness graft and suture it in place. Any adherent fat and as much cornified epithelium as possible must be cut and scraped away using a scalpel blade. This will produce a thinner, more pliable graft that will have much less tendency to lift off its underlying granulation bed as the cornified epithelium dries and contracts. Leaving long ends on the sutures will allow you to tie on a compressive pad that

will help prevent fluid accumulation under the graft. A simple finger tip compression dressing can serve the same purpose.

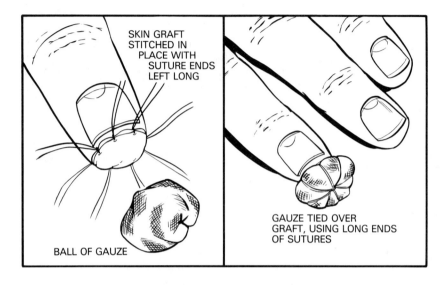

SKIN GRAFT
STITCHED IN
PLACE WITH
SUTURE ENDS
LEFT LONG

BALL OF GAUZE

GAUZE TIED OVER
GRAFT, USING LONG ENDS
OF SUTURES

c) With a large area of tissue loss that has been thoroughly cleaned and debrided and where the avulsed portion has been lost or destroyed, consider a thin split-thickness skin graft on the site. Using 1% Xylocaine, raise an intradermal wheal on the volar aspect of the patient's wrist until it is the size of a quarter. Then, with a #10 scalpel blade, slice off a very thin graft from this site. Apply the graft in the same manner as the full thickness one (above) with a compression dressing.

• A dressing change should be arranged in 4 days. During that time the patient should be instructed to keep his finger elevated and at rest.

• If an associated fracture is present, apply a protective splint and start prophylactic antibiotics.

What not to do:

• Do not apply a graft directly over bone or over a potentially devitalized or contaminated bed.

Discussion:

Treating small and medium-sized finger tip amputations without grafting is becoming increasingly popular. Allowing repair by wound contracture may leave the patient with as good a result and possibly better sensation, without the discomfort or minor disfigurement of taking a split thickness graft. On the other hand, covering the site with a graft may give the patient a more useful and less sensitive fingertip within a shorter period of time. Unlike the full-thickness graft, a thin split-thickness graft will allow wound contracture and thereby allow for skin with normal sensitivity to be drawn over the end of the finger. The full-thickness graft, on the other hand, will give an early, tough cover which is insensitive but has a more normal appearance. The technique followed should be determined by the nature of the wound as well as the special occupational and emotional needs of the patient. Explain these options to the patient, who can help decide your course of action.

Nail Root Dislocation

Presentation:

The patient will most likely have dropped a heavy object like a can of vegetables on a bare toe, with the edge of the can striking the base of the toenail and causing a painful deformity. The base of the nail will be found resting above the eponychium instead of in its anatomical position beneath it. The cuticular line that had joined the eponychium at the nail fold will remain attached to the nail at its original position.

What to do:

- X ray to rule out an underlying fracture (which would require a prophylactic antibiotic as well as protective splinting.)
- Anesthetize the area using a digital block. (See p 283.)
- Lift the base of the nail off the eponychium, and thoroughly cleanse, debride, and inspect the nail bed.
- Repair any nailbed lacerations with a fine absorbable suture (7–0 Vicryl).
- Reinsert the root of the nail under the eponychium.
- Reduce any underlying angulated fracture.
- If the nail tends to drift out from under the eponychium, it can be sutured in place. Sutures should be removed after one week.
- Cover the area with a finger tip dressing and splint any underlying fracture.
- Provide tetanus prophylaxis.
- Followup should be provided in 3–5 days.

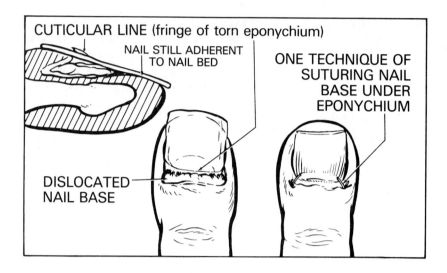

CUTICULAR LINE (fringe of torn eponychium)

NAIL STILL ADHERENT TO NAIL BED

ONE TECHNIQUE OF SUTURING NAIL BASE UNDER EPONYCHIUM

DISLOCATED NAIL BASE

What not to do:

- Do not ignore the nail root dislocation and simply provide a finger tip dressing. This is likely to lead to continued bleeding or to a later infection because tissue planes have not been replaced in their natural anatomic position.
- Do not dispose of the nail unless it is significantly damaged or contaminated. This nail will provide the most comfortable fingertip dressing.

Discussion:

It may be surprising that this injury is often missed but at first glance, a dislocated nail can appear to be in place, and without careful inspection, a patient can return from radiology with negative x rays and be treated as if he only had an abrasion/contusion.

The attachment of the cuticle from the nailfold of the eponychium to the base of the nail forms a constant landmark on the nail. If any nail is showing proximal to this landmark it indicates that the nail is not in its normal position beneath the eponychium.

Fingernail or Toenail Avulsion

Presentation:

The patient may have had a blow to the nail; the nail may have been torn away by a fan blade or other piece of machinery; or a long hard toenail may have caught on a loop of a shag carpet or other fixed object and been pulled off the nailbed.

The nail may be completely avulsed, partially held in place by the nail folds, or adhering only to the distal nail bed. On occasion, an exposed nailbed will have a pearly appearance with minimal bleeding making it seem as if the nail is still in place when actually it has been completely avulsed.

What to do:

- Obtain x rays if there was any crushing or high velocity shearing force involved.
- Perform a digital block to anesthetize the entire nailbed (see p 283).
- Cleanse the nailbed with normal saline and remove any loose cuticular debris. Although it is acceptable simply to cover the nailbed with a non-adherent dressing, the patient is usually more comfortable with a clean nail or surrogate in place while a new nail grows in.
- If the nail is still tenuously attached, remove it by separating it from the nailfold using a hemostat. Cleanse the nail thoroughly with normal saline, cut away the distal portion of the nail and remove adherent cuticular debris.
- Reinsert the nail under the eponychium and apply a fingertip dressing (see Appendix).
- If the nail is missing, badly damaged or contaminated, replace it with a substitute. An artificial nail can be cut out of the sterile aluminum foil found in a suture pack or can be cut from a sheet of vaseline gauze. Insert this stent under the eponychium as you would the nail and apply a fingertip dressing after it is in place.

    Leave these stents in place until the nailbed hardens and the stent separates spontaneously. Dressings should be changed every three to five days.

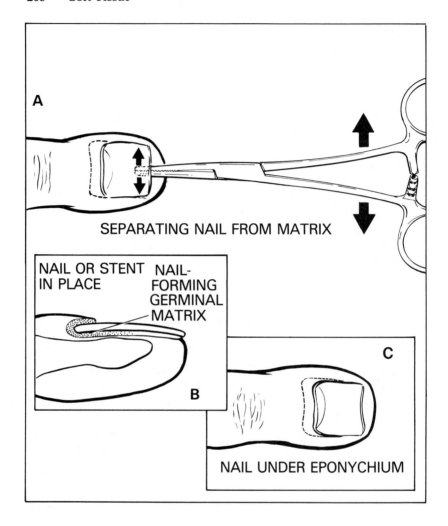

A

SEPARATING NAIL FROM MATRIX

NAIL OR STENT   NAIL-
IN PLACE   FORMING
                GERMINAL
                MATRIX

B

C

NAIL UNDER EPONYCHIUM

What not to do:

- Do not dress an exposed nailbed with an ordinary gauze dressing. It will adhere to the nailbed and require lengthy soaks and at times an extremely painful removal.
- Do not ignore nailbed lacerations or fractures of the distal phalanx. The new nail can become deformed or ingrown wherever the bed is not smooth and straight.

Discussion:

Although the eponychium is unlikely to scar to the nailbed unless there is infection, inflammation, or considerable tissue damage, separating the eponychium from the nail matrix by reinserting the nail or inserting an artificial stent helps to prevent synechia and future nail deformities from developing. The patient's own nail is also his most comfortable dressing.

Ring Removal

Presentation:

A ring has become tight on the patient's finger after an injury (usually a sprain of the PIP joint) or after some other cause of swelling, such as a local reaction to a bee sting. Sometimes, tight-fitting rings obstruct lymphatic drainage, causing swelling and further constriction. The patient usually wants the ring removed even if it requires cutting it off, but occasionally a patient has a very personal attachment to the ring and objects to its cutting or removal.

What to do:

- Limit further swelling by applying ice and elevating the extremity.
- When a fracture is suspected, order appropriate x rays either before or after removing the ring.
- With substantial injuries, a digital or metacarpal block might be necessary to allow for the comfortable removal of the ring.
- Most commonly, lubrication with soap and water along with proximal traction on the skin beneath the ring is enough to help you twist the ring off the finger.
- When the ring is too tight to twist off this way, exsanguinate the finger by applying a tightly wrapped spiral of Penrose drain around the exposed portion of the finger, elevate the hand above the head, wait five minutes and then apply a BP cuff inflated to 200mm Hg as a tourniquet around the upper arm. Then, remove the Penrose drain and, leaving the tourniquet in place, again attempt to twist the ring off using soap and water for lubrication.
- If the ring is still too tight or there is too much pain to allow for the above techniques, a ring cutter can be used to cut through a narrow ring band. Bend the ring apart with pliers placed on either side of this break to complete removal.
- If the band is wide or made of hard metal, it will be much easier

to cut out a 5mm wedge from the ring using an orthopedic pin cutter. Then take a cast spreader, place it in the groove formed by the removal of the wedge and spread the ring apart like a clam shell. Alternatively, two cuts may be made on opposite sides of the ring, allowing it to be removed in halves.

- Another useful device for removing constricting metal bands is the Dremel Moto-tool with its sharp-edged grinder attachment.*

- Another technique which tends to be rather time-consuming and only moderately effective (but one that can be readily attempted in the field) is the coiled string technique. Slip the end of a string (kite string would be a good example) under the ring and wind a tight single-layer coil down the finger, compressing the swelling as you go. Pull up on the end of the string under the ring, then slide and wiggle the ring down over the coil. (In the case of a sprain of the PIP joint, this technique may cause considerable discomfort.)

- Teach patients how to avoid the vicious cycle of a tourniquet effect by promptly removing rings from injured fingers.

What not to do:

- When a patient is expected to have transient swelling of the hand or finger without evidence of vascular compromise, and he requests that the ring not be removed, do not be insistent that you must cut the ring off. If the patient is at all responsible, he can be warned of vascular compromise (pallor, cyanosis, or pain) and instructed to keep his hand elevated and apply cool compresses. He should then be made to understand that he is to return for further care if the circulation does become compromised because of the possible risk of losing his finger. Be understanding and document the patient's request and your directions.

Discussion:

The constricting effects of a circumferential foreign body can lead to obstruction of lymphatic drainage, which in turn leads to more swelling and further constriction, until venous and eventually arterial circulation is compromised. If you believe that these consequences are inevitable you should be quite direct with the patient about having the ring removed.

---

*Greenspan L: Tourniquet syndrome caused by metallic bands: a new tool for removal. Ann Emerg Med 1982; 11:375–378.

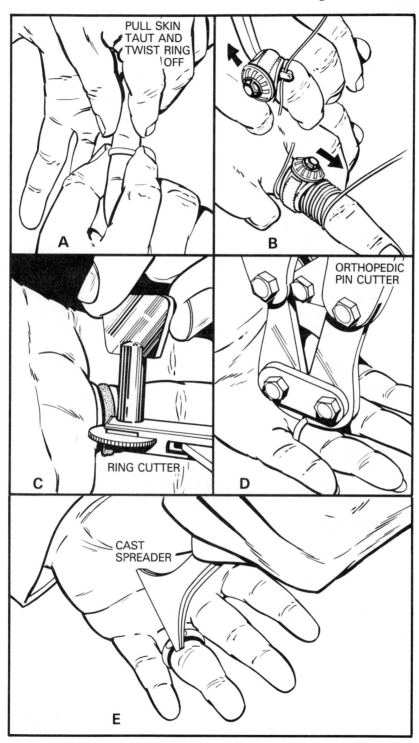

PULL SKIN TAUT AND TWIST RING OFF

A

B

RING CUTTER

C

ORTHOPEDIC PIN CUTTER

D

CAST SPREADER

E

Nailbed Laceration

Presentation:

The patient will have either cut into his nailbed with a sharp edge or crushed his finger. With shearing forces, the nail may be avulsed from the nailbed to varying degrees and there may be an underlying bony deformity.

What to do:

- Provide appropriate tetanus prophylaxis.
- Obtain x rays of any crush injury.
- Perform a digital block for anesthesia (see Appendix).
- With a simple laceration through the nail, remove the nail surrounding the laceration to allow for suturing the laceration closed:
    a) Use a straight hemostat to separate the nail from the nailbed.
    b) Use fine scissors to cut away the surrounding nail.
    c) Cleanse the wound with saline and suture with a fine absorbable suture (7–0 Vicryl or Dexon).
    d) Apply a nonadherent dressing (e.g., Adaptic gauze) and antibiotic antiseptic ointment and plan a dressing change within 24 hours to prevent painful adherence to the nailbed.

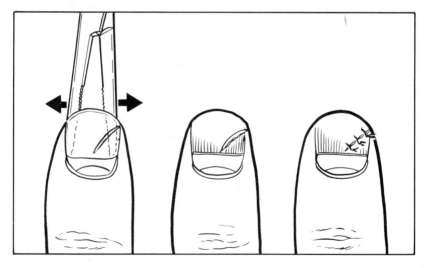

- When a crush injury results in open hemorrhage from under the fingernail, the nail must be completely elevated to allow proper inspection of the damage to the nailbed. A bloodless field helps visualization. (A one half-inch Penrose drain makes a good finger tourniquet.) Angulated fractures need to be reduced and nailbed lacerations should be sutured with a fine absorbable suture (7–0 Vicryl or Dexon). The nail can be cleaned and re-inserted for protection or a nailbed dressing can be applied.

What not to do:

- Do not use non-absorbable sutures to repair the nailbed. The patient will be put through unnecessary suffering in order to remove the sutures.
- Do not attempt to suture a nailbed laceration through the nail. It can be done, but precludes the meticulous approximation necessary for smooth nail regrowth.

Discussion:

Significant nailbed injuries can be hidden by hemorrhage and a partially avulsed overlying nail. These injuries must be repaired to help prevent future deformity of the nail.

Surgical consultation should be obtained when nailbed lacerations involve the germinal matrix under the base of the nail.

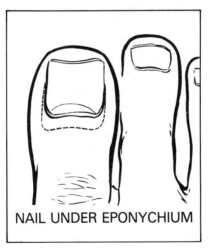

NAIL UNDER EPONYCHIUM

Subungual Hematoma

Presentation:

After a blow or crushing injury to the fingernail, the patient experiences severe and sometimes excruciating pain, that persists for hours, and may even be associated with a vaso-vagal response. The fingernail has an underlying deep blue-black discoloration which may be localized to the proximal portion of the nail or extend beneath its entire surface.

What to do:

- X ray the finger to rule out an underlying fracture of the distal phalanx.
- Paint the nail with Betadine.
- Perform a trephination at the base of the nail, using a hot paper clip, electric cauterizing lance or drill.
- Have the patient hold a folded 4″ × 4″ gauze pad firmly over the trephination while holding his hands over his head until the bleeding stops.
- Apply an antibacterial ointment such as Betadine and cover the trephination with a Band-Aid.
- To prevent infection, instruct the patient to keep his finger dry for 2 days and not to soak it (e.g., go swimming) for 1 week.
- If there is an underlying fracture, the patient should be instructed to keep his finger completely dry for the next ten days and should also be placed on a short course of antibiotics. (Keflex 500mg qid x 4d).
- A protective aluminum finger tip splint may also be comforting.
- Inform the patient that he will eventually lose his fingernail, until a new nail grows out after several months.

What not to do:

- Do not perform a trephination on a subungual ecchymosis (see p 216).
- Do not perform a trephination when there is an underlying fracture (this theoretically converts a closed fracture to an open one) unless there is sufficient pain to justify it. The patient should also understand the potential risk of developing osteomyelitis, as well as the need for keeping the finger dry.
- Do not perform a trephination on a patient who is no longer experiencing any significant pain at rest. A mild analgesic and a protective splint will usually suffice.

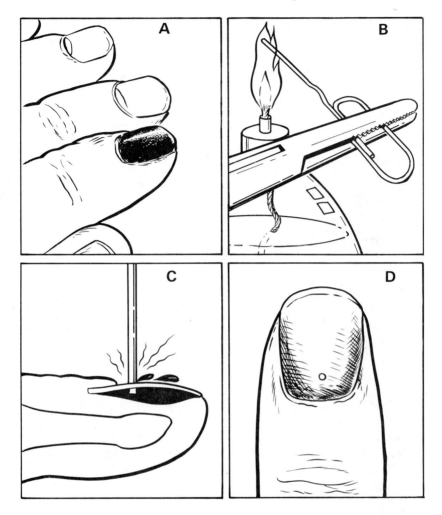

- Do not send a patient home to soak his finger after a trephination. This will break down the protective fibrin clot and introduce bacteria into this previously sterile space.

Discussion:

The subungual hematoma is a space-occupying mass that produces pain secondary to increased pressure against the very sensitive nailbed and matrix. Given time, the tissues surrounding this collection of blood will stretch and deform until the pressure within this mass equilibrates. Within 24 hours the pain therefore subsides and, although the patient may continue to complain of pain with activity, performing a trephination at this time will not improve his discomfort to any significant extent and will expose the patient to the risk of infection. If you choose not to perform a trephination, explain your reason, so a patient who is aware of such a procedure doesn't assume that you don't know what you're doing.

Subungual Ecchymosis

Presentation:

The patient will have had a crushing injury over the fingernail; getting it caught between two heavy objects for example, or striking it with a hammer. The pain is initially intense, but rapidly subsides over the first half hour, and by the time he is examined only mild pain and sensitivity may remain. There is a light brown or light blue-brown discoloration beneath the nail.

What to do:

- Get an x ray to rule out a possible fracture of the distal phalangeal tuft.
- Apply a protective fingertip splint, if necessary for comfort.
- Explain why you are not drilling a hole in the patient's nail, and inform the patient that, in time, he may lose the fingernail; a new nail will replace it.

What not to do:

- Do not perform a trephination of the nail.

Discussion:

Unlike the painful space-occupying subungual hematoma, the subungual ecchymosis only represents a thin extravasation of blood beneath the nail or a mild separation of the nail from the nailbed. Doing a trephination will not relieve any pressure or pain, and may indeed cause excruciating pain, as well as open this space to possible infection. The general public's familiarity with nail trephination may give the patient the erroneous expectation that he should have his nail drilled. Therefore, he will require an explanation as to why it is not indicated under these circumstances if he is to leave your department satisfied and reassured.

Foreign Body Beneath Nail

Presentation:

The patient complains of a paint chip or sliver under the nail. Often he has unsuccessfully attempted to remove the foreign body, which will be visible beneath the nail.

What to do: (Paint Chip)

- Without anesthesia, remove overlying nail by shaving it with a #15 scalpel blade.
- Cleanse remaining debris with normal saline and trim the nail edges smooth with scissors.
- Provide tetanus prophylaxis if necessary and then dress the area with antibiotic ointment and a bandage.

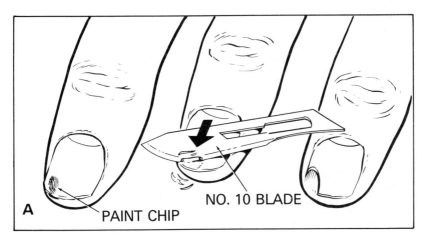

A PAINT CHIP NO. 10 BLADE

What to do: (Sliver)

- If the patient is cooperative and can tolerate some discomfort, carve through the nail down to the perimeter of the sliver with a #11 blade until the overlying nail falls away. The FB can now be cleansed away, antibiotic ointment can be applied to the exposed nailbed, and a Band-Aid dressing can be applied.
- For a more extensive excision of a nail wedge, you will need to perform a digital block (see Appendix).
- Slide small Mayo scissors between the nail and nailbed on both sides of the sliver and cut out the overlying wedge of nail.
- Cleanse any remaining debris with normal saline and trim the fingernail until the corners are smooth.

- Provide tetanus prophylaxis if needed (see p 277).
- Dress with antibiotic ointment and a bandage. Have the patient redress the area 2–3 times daily until healed, and keep the fingernail trimmed close.

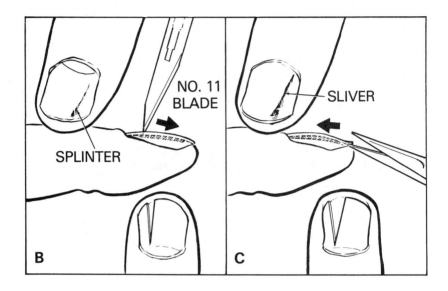

What not to do:

- Do not run the tip of the scissors into the nailbed while sliding it under fingernail (instead angle the tip up into undersurface of the nail).

Discussion:

It is often not possible to remove a long sliver from beneath the fingernail using the "shaving" technique with a scapel blade, without injuring the nailbed, and causing the patient considerable discomfort.

After providing a digital block, it is sometimes possible to remove the sliver by surrounding it with a hemostat that has been slipped between the nail and nailbed and then pulling out the entire sliver, but if any debris remains visible, then the overlying nail wedge should be removed.

It is usually unwise simply to attempt to pull the foreign body from beneath the nail because some debris usually remains and will most likely lead to a nailbed infection.

Paronychia

Presentation:

The patient will come with finger or toe pain that is either chronic and recurrent in nature or has developed rapidly over the past several hours, accompanied by redness and swelling of the nail fold. There are three distinct varieties.

The chronic paronychia is most commonly seen with the "ingrown toenail" with chronic inflammation, thickening and purulence of the eponychial fold and loss of the cuticle. This also occurs with individuals whose hands are frequently macerated.

The acute paronychia is much more painful and is caused by the introduction of pyogenic bacteria by minor trauma resulting in acute inflammation and abscess formation within the thin subcutaneous layer between the skin of the eponychial fold and the germinal layer of the eponychial cul-de-sac.

The third variety of paronychia is a subungual abscess, which occurs in the same location as a subungual hematoma, between the nail plate and the nail bed.

What to do:

- Perform a unilateral or bilateral digital block if a significant surgical procedure is anticipated (see Appendix).
- With a chronic paronychia:
  a) You may consider conservative treatment or temporizing the condition by sliding a cotton wedge under the corner of an ingrown nail and placing the patient on antibiotics (e.g., Cefadroxil (Duricef) 1gm qid and warm soaks. When candidiasis is suspected, the area should be kept dry and treated with local applications of nystatin. Surgical followup is important.
  b) A more aggressive approach, and one more likely to be successful, is to sharply excise the affected portion of the nail, nailbed and matrix down to the periosteum of the distal phalynx. The patient is instructed to soak the toe in warm soapy water for 20 min bid.
- With an acute paronychia:
  a) Taking an 18 gauge needle or #15 scalpel blade, *separate* the cuticle from the nail thereby opening the eponychial cul-de-sac and draining any abscess. There is no need actually to make an incision and therefore a digital block should not be necessary. A tiny wick (1cm of ¼" gauze) may be slid into the opening to ensure continued drainage.

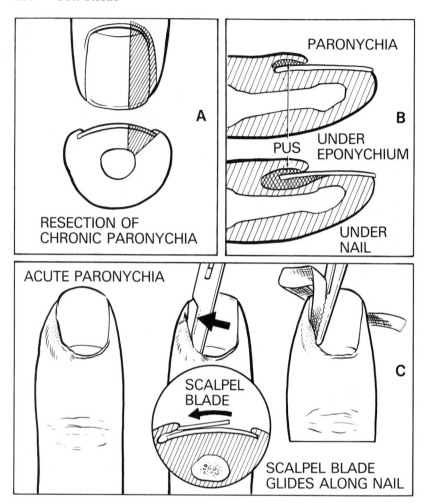

This technique will require frequent warm soaks (at least qid) and, where significant cellulitis was present, a short course of antibiotics (e.g., Duricef 1gm qid x 3–4d) may be indicated. The patient should be informed that if the paronychia quickly recurs, excision of a portion of the nail might be required.

b) A more aggressive approach is to excise a portion of the nail. Unlike the more extensive procedure used with the chronic paronychia only a portion of the nail need be removed. After digital block, simply insert a fine straight hemostat between the nail and the nail bed and push and spread until you enter the eponychia cul-de-sac. Often it is at this point that pus is discovered. Then using a pair of fine scissors, cut away ¼–⅓ of the nail bordering the paronychia. Separate the cuticle using the hemostat and pull this unwanted fragment away. A non-adherent dressing is required over the exposed nailbed as well as an early dressing change (within 48 hours).

- With a subungual abscess:
  a) You may consider conservative treatment not requiring a digital block. Merely perform a trephination using the same "hot paper clip" technique used for a subungual hematoma. The patient must provide frequent warm soapy soaks over the next 36 hours to prevent recurrence. An antibiotic such as Duricef may also be helpful.
  b) The more effective but more aggressive technique requires removal of the proximal ⅓ of the the nail. A straight hemostat is required to separate the cuticle of the eponychium from the underlying nail. Using the hemostat, the proximal portion of the nail is pulled out from under the eponychium and excised. On occasion an incision will have to be made along the eponychium to allow the proximal nail to be excised.

  The removal of the proximal portion of the nail allows for the complete drainage of the abscess without any risk of recurrence. A non-adherent dressing is also required in this instance. Extensive damage to the germinal matrix by the infection may preclude healthy nail regrowth.

What not to do:

- Do not remove an entire fingernail or toenail to drain a simple paronychia.
- Do not confuse a felon (tense tender finger pad) with a paronychia. Felons will require more extensive surgical treatment.

Discussion:

Whenever conservative therapy is instituted, the patient should be advised as to the advantages and disadvantages of that approach. If your patient is not willing or reliable enough to perform the required aftercare or cannot accept the potential treatment failure, then it would seem prudent to begin with the more aggressive treatment modes.

Bicycle Spoke Injury

Presentation:

A small child, riding on the back of a friend's bike, gets his foot caught between the spinning spokes and the frame or fender supports. The skin over the lateral or medial aspect of the foot or ankle is crushed and abraded with underlying soft tissue swelling.

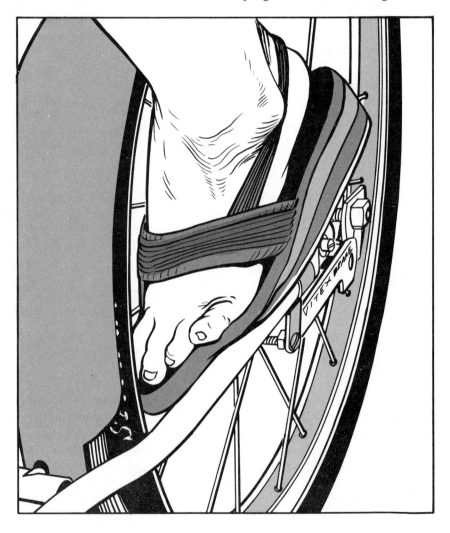

What to do:

- Cleanse the area with a gentle scrub (Betadine).
- Provide any tetanus prophylaxis required and apply a tempo-

rary normal saline dressing.

- Get radiographic studies to rule out any fracture.
- Dress the wound with povodone iodine (Betadine) ointment and a non-adherent cover such as Adaptic gauze. Incorporate a bulky compressive dressing consisting of gauze fluffs, Kerlex and a mildly compressive ACE wrap.
- Have the patient keep the foot strictly elevated over the next 24 hours and schedule him for a wound check within 48 hours.
- Inform the parents that the crushed skin is not a simple abrasion and may not survive. They should understand that a slow-healing sore might result or skin grafting might be required, and therefore careful surgical followup is necessary.

What not to do:

- Do not assume that because the x rays are negative you are merely dealing with a simple abrasion.

Discussion:

Bicycle spoke injuries are similar to, but not as serious as, wringer injuries. Fractures are not commonly associated with these injuries but often there is severe soft tissue injury. Consequences of this crush injury can be minimized by the use of compression dressings, elevation and early followup.

Needle (Foreign Body) in Foot

Presentation:

Although a needle could be embedded under any skin surface, most commonly a patient will have stepped on one while running or sliding barefoot on a carpeted floor. Generally, but not invariably, the patient will complain of a foreign body sensation with weight bearing. A very small puncture wound will be found at the point of entry, and, on occasion, a portion of the needle will be palpable beneath the skin.

What to do:

- Tape a partially opened paper clip as a skin marker to the plantar surface of the foot, with the tip of the opened paper clip over the entrance wound. Instruct the patient not to allow

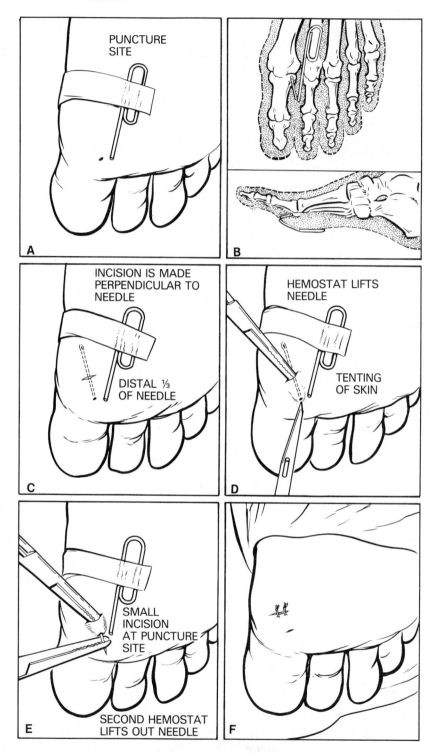

A PUNCTURE SITE

B

C INCISION IS MADE PERPENDICULAR TO NEEDLE DISTAL ⅓ OF NEEDLE

D HEMOSTAT LIFTS NEEDLE TENTING OF SKIN

E SMALL INCISION AT PUNCTURE SITE SECOND HEMOSTAT LIFTS OUT NEEDLE

F

anyone to remove the paper clip until after the needle is removed.

- Send the patient for PA and lateral radiographs of the foot with the skin marker in place.
- Evaluate the x rays. If the needle appears to be very deep you may choose to call in a consultant who can remove the needle under fluoroscopy. If the needle is relatively superficial, inform the patient that removing a needle is not as easy as it appears. Let him know that you are going to use a simple technique for locating and removing the needle, but that sometimes the needle is hidden within the tissue of the foot ("like a needle in a haystack"). If you cannot locate the needle within 10–15 minutes, because you do not want to further damage his foot, you will call in a consultant or arrange for fluoroscopy.
- Establish a bloodless field by elevating the leg above the level of the heart, tightly wrapping an ACE bandage around the foot and lower leg, and then inflating and clamping off a thigh cuff at approximately 200mmHg. This will become uncomfortable within 10–15 minutes and thereby serve as an automatic timer for your procedure.
- Remove the ACE wrap, clean and then paint the area with Betadine solution, and locally infiltrate the appropriate area with plain 1% Xylocaine. (It will be somewhat more comfortable if the needle stick is accomplished from the medial or lateral aspect of the foot rather than directly into the plantar surface.)
- The x rays should give you an idea of the location of the needle relative to the paper clip skin marker.
- With the patient lying prone and the plantar surface of his foot facing upward, make an incision that crosses perpendicular to the needle's apparent position at its midpoint or ⅓ of the way toward the most superficial end of the needle. Do not cut deep to the plantar fascia.

- As you cut across the needle, there will be an audible clicking sound. Spread the incision apart, visualize the needle and grasp it firmly with a hemostat or small Kelly clamp.
- Now, push the needle out in the direction from which it entered. Even the eye or back end of a broken needle is sharp enough to be pushed to the skin surface. If the needle tents up the skin and will not push through, nick the overlying skin surface with a scalpel blade until the needle exits. Grab this end with another clamp, let go with the first clamp, and remove the needle.

- Let the thigh cuff down and suture your incision closed. Apply an appropriate dressing.
- Provide tetanus prophylaxis indicated.

What not to do:

- Do not ignore the patient who thinks he stepped on a needle but in whom you can't find a puncture wound. Get an x ray anyway because the puncture wound is probably hidden.
- Do not give the patient the impression that the removal will be quick and easy. You will be setting yourself up for an embarrassing failure.
- Do not make your incision near the tip of the needle or directly over and parallel to the needle. The needle will not be exactly where you think it is, and your incision will miss exposing the needle.
- Do not persist in extensively undermining or extending your incision if you do not locate the needle within 10 minutes of beginning the procedure. This is unlikely to be productive and you may do the patient harm.
- Do not routinely place the patient on prophylactic antibiotics. They are unnecessary.
- Do not attempt to remove a needle by pulling on the attached thread. It usually breaks, and may create a second foreign body to remove.

Discussion:

Many a young doctor has been found sweating away at the foot of an emergency department stretcher, unable to locate a needle foreign body. The secret for improving your chances of success is in realizing that the x ray only gives you an *approximate* location of the needle and that your incision must be made in a direction and location best suited for *locating* the needle, not *removing* it.

When you let the patient know how difficult it sometimes is to locate the needle and remove it, you place yourself in a win-win situation. You look especially good if you find it and you still look experienced and well-informed if you don't.

If you choose to take the patient to fluoroscopy, you or the radiologist can place a hemostat around the needle under direct vision. It can then be pushed out using the same technique described above.

Puncture Wounds

Presentation:

Most commonly, the patient will have stepped or jumped onto a nail. The patient is often only asking for a tetanus shot and can usually be found in the emergency department with his foot soaking in a basin of Betadine solution. The wound entrance usually appears as a stellate tear in the cornified epithelium on the plantar surface of the foot.

What to do:

- Obtain a detailed history to ascertain the force involved in creating the puncture and the relative cleanliness of the penetrating object.
- Examine the foot for signs of deep injury such as swelling and pain with motion of the toes. Although the occurrence is unlikely, test for loss of sensory or motor function.
- With deep, highly contaminated wounds, orthopedic consultation should be sought to consider a wide debridement in the operating room. This is done to prevent the catastrophic complication of osteomyelitis. Most puncture wounds only require simple debridement and irrigation.
- Saucerize the puncture wound using a #10 scalpel blade to remove the cornified epithelium and any debris that has collected beneath its surface.
- If debris is found, gently slide a large-gauge needle (preferably blunt) or an Angiocath catheter down the wound track and slowly irrigate with a physiologic saline solution until debris no longer flows from the wound. At times, a small amount of local anesthesia will be necessary to accomplish this.
- For other than small, clean puncture wounds, prescribe a prophylactic antibiotic, (e.g., Cefadroxil 1gm qid x 4). Tetanus prophylaxis should be provided for all wounds.
- Cover the wound with a Band-Aid and instruct the patient on the warning signs of infection.

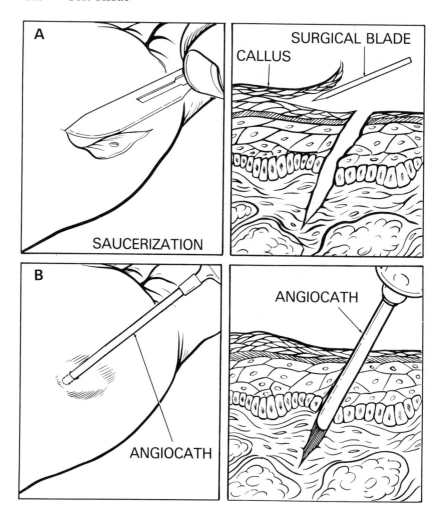

What not to do:

- Do not be falsely reassured by having the patient soak in Betadine. This does not provide any significant protection from infection and is not a substitute for debridement (saucerization) and irrigation.
- Do not attempt a jet lavage within a puncture wound. This will only lead to subcutaneous infiltration of your irrigant.
- Do not get x rays except for the unusual case where large particulate debris is suspected to be deeply imbedded within the wound.
- Do not begin soaks at home unless there are early signs of infection developing.

Discussion:

It should be understood that the only usefulness of Betadine soaks is to give the patient, who is awaiting his turn to be seen, the feeling that something is being done for him.

When the foot is punctured, the cornified epithelium acts as a spatula, cleaning off any loose material from the penetrating object as it slides by. This debris often collects just beneath this cornified layer which then acts like a trap door holding it in. Left in place, this debris normally leads to early abscess formation. Saucerization will allow removal of the debris as well as elimination of the trap door effect, in the event that infection develops and drainage is required. Saucerization can also be useful for unroofing small foreign bodies or abscesses found beneath thickly cornified skin surfaces.

Puncture wounds that are caused by friable, radiopaque material like glass should be x rayed to rule out a possible foreign body.

Minor Impalement Injuries

Presentation:

A sharp metal object such as a needle, heavy wire, nail or fork is driven into or through a patient's extremity. In some instances, the patient may arrive with a large object attached; for instance, a child who has stepped on a nail going through a board. As minor as most of these injuries are, they tend to create a spectacle and draw a crowd.

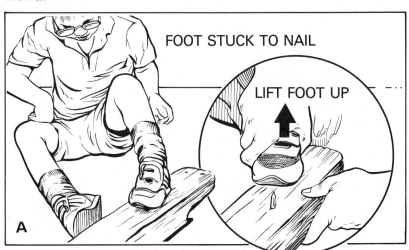

FOOT STUCK TO NAIL

LIFT FOOT UP

A

What to do:

- If you are dealing with an impaled object attached to something that is acting like a lever and causing pain with any movement (as with the case of the child above), either *quickly* cut off this lever or immediately pull the patient's extremity off the sharp object. (You can usually cut a nail or metal spike with an orthopedic pin cutter.)

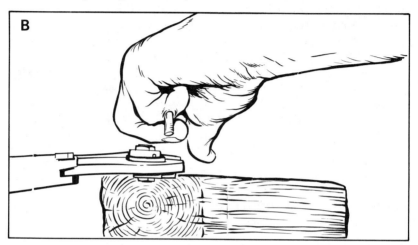

- X rays should be obtained when pain and further damage from a leveraged object is not a problem, and when there is a suspicion of an underlying fracture, fragmentation, or hooking of the impaled object, as might occur with a heavy wire that has been thrown from under a lawnmower.
- Examine the extremity for possible neurovascular or tendon injury.
- If surgical debridement is anticipated after removal of the object, then infiltration of an anesthetic should be provided prior to removal. Otherwise, consider whether or not the patient wants a shot of local anesthetic before the object is quickly pulled out. Local anesthesia will usually not give complete pain relief when a deeply imbedded object is removed; inform the patient of this.
- Fishhook—see p 231.
- Objects with small barbs, such as crochet needles and fish spines, can be removed by first anesthetizing the area and then applying firm traction until the barb is revealed through the puncture wound. The fibrils of connective tissue caught over the barb can then be cut with a scalpel blade or fine scissors.

- After removal of the impaled object the wound should be appropriately debrided and irrigated. Tetanus prophylaxis should be provided and, except for small, clean wounds, a prophylactic antibiotic should be prescribed (e.g., Duricef 1gm qid x 4d).

What not to do:

- Do not send a patient to x ray with a leveraged object impaled, creating further pain and possible injury with every movement.
- Do not try to hand-saw off a board attached to an impaled object. The resultant movement will obviously cause unnecessary pain and possibly harm.

Discussion:

Simple impalement injuries of the extremities should not be confused with major impalement injuries of the neck and trunk in which the foreign object usually should *not* be precipitously removed. With major impalement injuries careful localization with x rays is required, and full exposure and vascular control in the operating room is also a necessity to prevent rapid exsanguination when the impaled object is removed from the heart or a great vessel.

Fishhook Removal

Presentation:

The patient has been snagged with a fishhook and arrives with it embedded in his skin.

What to do:

- If a multifaceted (treble) hook is embedded, use a pin cutter or metal snips to remove the free hooks and protect the patient as well as yourself from additional harm. When significant manipulation is anticipated, infiltrate first with 1% lidocaine.
- When a single hook is embedded in a stable skin surface such as the back, scalp or arm, the best way to remove it is by using a simple string technique. Align the shaft of the hook so that it is parallel to skin surface. Press down on the hook with your index finger to disengage the barb. Place a loop of string (fishing line or 1–0 silk) over your wrist and around the hook, and with a

quick jerk opposite from the direction the shaft of the hook is running, pop the hook out. When done properly, this procedure is painless and does not require anesthesia.

- "Needling" the hook is an alternative technique that requires somewhat greater skill but allows you to work on an unstable skin surface such as a finger or ear. Slide a large gauge (#20 or #18) hypodermic needle through the wound alongside the hook. Now blindly slide the needle opening over the barb of the hook and, holding the hook firmly, lock the two together. Now, with the barb covered, remove the hook and needle as one unit. Since the needle does not cut through the dermis, there is usually no need for local anesthesia.

  With a hook that is superficially embedded, the needle may be used as a miniature scalpel blade. You can manipulate the hook into a position that will allow you to cut the bands of connective tissue caught over the barb, thereby releasing the hook. Gentle movement of the hook will often be interpreted by the patient as being painful but in fact, if the patient is coached, he will usually be able to tolerate minor manipulations with only a local pulling sensation.

- When the hook is deeply embedded, or you are unable to utilize the previous techniques, proceed with the tried and true "push through" maneuver. Locally infiltrate the area with 1% lidocaine and then push the point of the hook along with its barb up through the skin. Now with a pin cutter or metal snip, cut off the tip of the hook and remove the shaft or cut off the shaft of the hook and pull the tip through.

What not to do:

- Do not try to remove a multiple hook or a fishing lure with more than one hook without first removing the free hooks.
- Do not attempt to use the "string" technique if the hook is near the patient's eye.

Discussion:

The quickest and easiest method for removing a fishhook is the string technique. This is the one technique you can use in the field because no special equipment or anesthesia is required. In addition there is no lengthening of the puncture track or creation of an additional puncture wound. This technique is not recommended when the hook is positioned on a skin surface that is likely to move when the string is pulled. This movement will cause the vector of force to change and therefore the barb may not release.

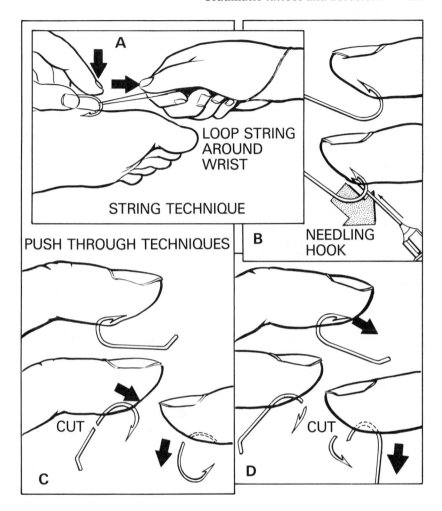

Traumatic Tattoos and Abrasions

Presentation:

The patient will usually have fallen onto a coarse surface such as a blacktop or macadam road. Most frequently, the skin of the face, forehead, chin, hands and knees are abraded. When pigmented foreign particles are impregnated within the dermis adventita, tattooing will occur. An explosive form of tattooing can also be seen with the use of firecrackers, firearms, and homemade bombs.

What to do:

- Cleanse the wound with nondestructive agents (e.g., normal saline,) and provide tetanus prophylaxis.
- With explosive tattooing, particles are generally deeply embedded and will require plastic surgical consultation. Any particles embedded in the dermis may become permanent "tattoos." Abrasions that are both large (more than several cm²) and uniformly deep into the dermis or below (so that no skin appendages, such as hair follicles, to provide a reservoir of regenerating basal epithelium remain), may also require consultation and/or skin grafts.
- With abrasions and abrasive tattooing, the area can usually be adequately anesthetised by applying 2% viscous Xylocaine or gauze soaked with TAC (tetracaine 0.5%, adrenaline 1:2000, and cocaine 11.8%) directly onto the wound for approximately 5 minutes. If this is not successful, locally infiltrate with 0.5% lidocaine with 1:200,000 epinephrine using a 25-gauge 3″ spinal needle for large areas.
- The wound should now be cleaned with a surgical scrub brush, saline and surgical soap. When impregnated material remains, use a sterile stiff toothbrush to clean the wound or use the side of a #10 scalpel blade to scrape away any debris. While working, continuously cleanse the wound surface with gauze soaked in normal saline to reveal any additional foreign particles. Large granules may be removed with the tip of a #11 blade.

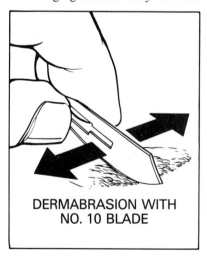

DERMABRASION WITH NO. 10 BLADE

- Wounds should be left open and povidone-iodine ointment applied. The patient should be instructed to gently wash the area 3–4 times per day and continue applying the ointment until the wound becomes dry and comfortable under a new coat of epithelium, which may require a few weeks.
- An alternative to the above when the wound has been adequately cleansed, is to use a closed dressing with Adaptic gauze and a scheduled dressing change within 2–3 days.

What not to do:

- Do not ignore embedded particles. If they cannot be completely

removed, inform the patient about the probability of permanent tattooing and arrange a plastic surgical consultation.

Discussion:

The technique of tattooing involves painting pigment on the skin,
and then injecting it through the epidermis into the dermis with a
needle. As the epidermis heals, the pigment particles are ingested
by macrophages and permanently bound into the dermis. Immediate care of traumatic tattoos is important because once the particles
are embedded and healing is complete, it becomes difficult to
remove them without scarring.

It is advisable for a patient to protect a dermabraded area from
sunlight for approximately 1 year to minimize excessive melaniza-
tion of the site.

Bites

Presentation:

Histories of animal bites are usually volunteered, but the history
of a human bite, such as one obtained over the knuckle during a
fight, is more likely to be denied or explained only after questioning.

A single bite may contain various types of injury, including
underlying fractures and tendon and nerve injuries. Not all of these
are immediately apparent.

What to do:

- A complete history should be obtained, including the type of
  animal involved, whether or not the attack was provoked, what
  time the injury occurred, the current health status and vaccination record of the animal, and whether or not the animal has
  been captured and is being held.
- If the wound requires debridement, or will be painful to cleanse
  and irrigate, anesthetize with plain Xylocaine (epinephrine
  slightly increases infection rates).
- Cleanse the wound with antiseptic (e.g., povidone-iodine,
  diluted 1:10 in normal saline), and sharply debride any debris
  and non-viable tissue.
- Irrigate the wound, using a 20ml syringe, a 19 gauge needle,
  and at least 200ml of sterile saline or the diluted povine-iodine

solution noted above. This technique demonstrably reduces microscopic debris and bacteria. Use an intravenous setup to irrigate a large area. Prepare every wound as if you were going to close it.

- For animal bite wounds that are lacerations located anywhere other than the hand or foot, you should staple, tape, or suture them closed.
- With human bites, or animal bites that are punctures, located on the hand or foot, or are more than 12 hours old, you should leave the wounds open and apply a light dressing. Wounds should also be left open on debilitated and immunocompromised patients.
- Start prophylactic antibiotics in the ED. The most effective dose is the one you can give now. Penicillin VK 500mg qid for 7–10 days should cover human and most animal mouth flora infections, including Pasteurella multocida, which occasionally is resistant to cephalosporins and semisynthetic penicillins. Use a penicillinase-resistant antibiotic like dicloxacillin 500mg qid if you are especially concerned about Staphylococcus aureus. Alternate antibiotic therapy could include cephalexin 500mg, po, qid (50–100mg/kg/day, four divided doses for children) or erythromycin 500mg qid (50mg/kg/day, four divided doses for children).
- If the patient has had no tetanus toxoid in the past 5–10 years, provide prophylaxis.
- If the patient was bitten by an oddly behaving domestic animal, or a bat, coyote, fox, opossum, raccoon, or skunk, you should start rapid rabies vaccination with 20IU/kg of rabies immune globulin and the first of five 1ml doses of human diploid strain rabies vaccine. Reassure the patient that bites of rodents and lagomorphs, including rats, squirrels, hamsters, and rabbits, in America do not usually transmit rabies (see p 278).
- Provide hepatitis prophylaxis for patients who have been bitten by known carriers of hepatitis B. Administer hepatitis B immune globulin 0.06ml/kg im at the time of injury and schedule a second dose in 30 days.
- Minimize edema (and infection) of hand wounds by splinting and elevation.
- Have patient return for a wound check in 2–3 days, or sooner if there is any sign of infection.

What not to do:

- Do not overlook a puncture wound.
- Do not suture debris, non-viable tissue, or a bacterial innoculum into a wound.

- Do not use buried absorbable sutures, which act as a foreign body and cause a reactive inflammation for about a month.
- Do not waste time and money obtaining cultures and Gram stains of fresh wounds. The results of these tests do not correlate well with the organisms that subsequently cause infection.

Discussion:

Animal bites are often brought promptly to the ED, if only because of a legal requirement to report the bite, or because of fear of rabies, justified or not. Human bites, on the other hand, are often not presented for care until they are infected, and the history must be suspected by the physician. For example, lacerations over the knuckles or excoriations on the penis may have actually been caused by teeth.

Animal bites occur most commonly among young, poorly supervised children who disturb the animals while they are sleeping or feeding, separate them during a fight, try to hug or kiss an unfamiliar animal or accidently frighten it. Less than 0.1% of all animal bites result in rabies.

Dog and cat bites both show high rates of infection with staphylococcus and streptococcus species, as well as *Pasteurella multocida* and many different gram-negative and anaerobic bacteria. In addition to these organisms, 10–30% of all human bites are infected with *Eikenella corrodens*, which sometimes show resistance to the semisynthetic penicillins, but sensitivity to penicillin. Adequate debridement and irrigation are clearly more effective than prophylactic antibiotics, and except in wounds that are at high risk for developing infection are often all that is required to prevent infection of bites.

For questions of local rabies risk, local public health services may be available and valuable support.

11

Skin

Rhus Dermatitis (Poison Ivy)

Presentation:

The patient is troubled with a pruritic rash made up of tense vesiculo-papular lesions on a mildly erythematous base. Typically these are found in groups of linear streaks and may be weeping, crusted, or confluent. If involvement is severe, there may be marked edema, particularly on the face and periorbital and genital areas. The thick protective stratum corneum of the palms and the soles generally protect these areas. The patient is often not aware of having been in contact with poison ivy, oak, or sumac but may recall working in a field or garden from 24–48 hours before the onset of symptoms.

What to do:

- Have the patient apply cool compresses of Burow's solution (Domeboro Powder Packets—2 pkts in 1 pint of water) for 20–30 minutes every 3–4 hours (more often if comforting).
- Small areas can be treated with topical steroids such as fluocinonide (Topsyn) gel 0.05% of betamethasone valerate cream 0.1% (Valisone) 2–3 times per day, enhanced at night with an occlusive plastic (Saran) wrap dressing.
- Hydroxyzine (Atarax) 25mg po q6h will help mild itching between application of compresses.
- Tepid tub baths with Aveeno colloidal oatmeal (1 cup in ½ tub) or cornstarch and baking soda (1 cup of each in ½ tub) will provide soothing relief.
- When severe reactions occur or in situations where the patient's livelihood is threatened, early and aggressive treatment with systemic corticosteroids should be initiated. Prednisone (60–80mg a day tapered over 2 weeks) will be necessary to prevent a later flare-up or rebound reaction. One 40mg dose of intramuscular triamcinolone acetonide (Kenalog) will be equally effective.

What not to do:

- Do not try to substitute pre-packaged steroid regimens (Medrol Dosepak, Aristopak). The course is not long enough and will lead to a flare up.
- Do not allow patients to apply fluorinated corticosteroids such as Topsyn or Valisone indefinitely to the face, where they can produce premature aging of the skin.
- Do not institute systemic steroids in the face of secondary infections such as impetigo, cellulitis, or erysipelas. Also, do not start steroids if there is a history of tuberculosis, diabetes, herpes or severe hypertension.

Discussion:

Poison oak and poison ivy are forms of allergic contact dermatitis that result from the exposure of sensitized individuals to allergens in sap. These allergens induce sensitization in more than 70 percent of the population, may be carried by pets, and are frequently transferred from hands to other areas of the body in the first few hours before the sap becomes fixed to the skin.

The gradual appearance of the eruption over a period of several days is a reflection of the amount of antigen deposited on the skin and the reactivity of the site, not an indication of any further spread of the allergen. The vesicle fluid is a transudate, does not contain antigen, and will not spread the eruption elsewhere on the body or to other people. The allergic skin reaction usually runs a course of about 2 weeks which is not shortened by any of the above treatments. The aim of therapy is to reduce the severity of symptoms, not to shorten the course.

Sunburn

Presentation:

Patients generally seek help only if their sunburn is severe. There will be a history of extended exposure to sunlight or to an artificial source of ultraviolet radiation, such as a sunlamp. The burns will be accompanied by intense pain and the patient will not be able to tolerate anything touching the skin. There may be systemic complaints that include nausea, chills, and fever. The affected areas are erythematous and are accompanied by mild edema. The more severe the burn, the earlier it will appear and the more likely it will progress to edema and blistering.

What to do:

- Inquire as to whether or not the patient is using a photosensitizing drug (e.g., tetracyclines, thiazides, sulfonamides, phenothiazines) and have the patient discontinue its use.
- Have the patient apply cool compresses of water or Burow's solution (Domeboro Powder Packets–1 pkt in 1 pint of water) as often as desired to relieve pain. This is the most comforting therapy.
- The patient may be helped by applying a topical steroid spray such as dexamethasone (Decaspray) and using an emollient such as Lubriderm.
- With a more severe burn prescribe a short course of systemic steroids (40–60mg of Prednisone qd x 3d). This will reduce inflammation, swelling, pain, and itching.

What not to do:

- Do not allow the patient to use OTC sunburn medications that contain local anesthetics (benzocaine, dibucaine or lidocaine). They are usually ineffective or only provide very transient relief. In addition there is the potential hazard of sensitizing the patient to these ingredients.
- Do not trouble the patient with unnecessary burn dressings. These wounds have a very low probability of becoming infected. Treatment should be directed at making the patient as comfortable as possible.

Discussion:

With sunburn, the onset of symptoms is usually delayed for 2–4 hours. Maximum discomfort usually occurs after 14–20 hours, and symptoms last between 24 and 72 hours. Patients should be instructed on the future use of sunscreens containing Para-aminobenzoic acid (PABA) (e.g., Pabanol and PreSun). Prophylactic use of aspirin prior to sun exposure has also been recommended.

Partial Thickness (Second-Degree) Burns and Tar Burns

Presentation:

Small, (<6% total body surface) partial thickness (second degree) burns can occur in a variety of ways. Spilled or splattered hot water and grease are among the most common causes, along with hot objects, explosive fumes, and burning (volatile) liquids. The patient will complain of excruciating pain and the burn will appear erythematous with vesicle formation. Some of these vesicles, or bullae, may have ruptured prior to the patient's arrival, while others may not develop for 24 hours. Tar burns are special in that tar adheres aggressively to the burned skin.

What to do:

- To stop the pain, immediately cover the burned area with sterile towels that have first been soaked in iced normal saline or an iced povidone-iodine solution. Continue irrigating the burn with the iced solution for the next 20–30 minutes or until the patient can remain comfortable without the cold compresses.
- Provide the patient with any necessary tetanus prophylaxis, and pain medication, (e.g., Percodan, Demerol).
- Examine the patient for any associated injuries and check the airway and pulmonary status of any patient with significant facial burns.
- When the pain has subsided, gently cleanse the burn with povidone-iodine scrub and rinse this off with normal saline.
- If the vesicles are not perforated, have a relatively thick wall, and are on a hairless surface such as the palm of the hand, they should be left intact. With small burns such as these, patients can be sent home to continue cold compresses for comfort. Otherwise, these vesicles should be protected from future rupture with a bulky sterile dressing.
- Open vesicles or bullae, large, thin-walled vesicles that are prone to rupture, or vesicles occurring on hairy surfaces that are prone to infection, should be completely debrided. Using fine scissors and forceps you can easily strip away any loose epithelium from the burn. (With tar burns, debridement should be accomplished in the same manner, removing the tar along with the loose epithelium. Tar adhering to normal epithelium can be left in place, acting as a sterile dressing in itself.)

  Rinse off any remaining debris with normal saline and cover all the open areas with an oil emulsion gauze (e.g., Adaptic) followed by silver sulfadiazene (Silvadene) cream and a bulky absorbent sterile dressing. The first dressing change should be scheduled in 2 days.

  Small burns and facial burns can often be treated with an open technique of using Silvadene cream only. Patients are instructed to wash the burn 4 times each day, followed by reapplication of the Silvadene cream.

Patients can be reassured that unless there are complications (such as infection) they do not have to worry about scarring.

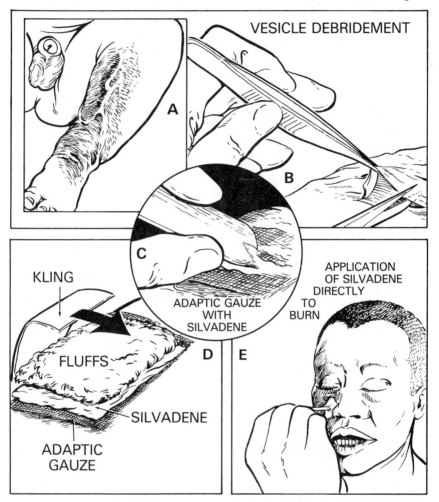

What not to do:

- Do not use ice-containing compresses which might increase tissue damage. Compresses soaked in iced saline should be avoided on large burns (greater than 15% total body surface) because they may lead to problems with hypothermia. When pain cannot be controlled with compresses use strong parenteral analgesics such as morphine sulfate.
- Do not confuse partial thickness burns with full thickness burns. Full thickness burns have no sensory function or skin appendages such as hair follicles remaining, do not form vesi-

cles, and may have evidence of thrombosed vessels. If areas of full thickness burn are present or suspected, seek surgical consultation because these areas will not grow new skin and may later require skin grafting.

- Do not discharge patients with suspected respiratory burns or extensive burns of the hands or genitalia. These patients require special inpatient observation and management.
- Do not use caustic solvents in an attempt to remove tar from burns. It is unnecessary, painful, and will cause further tissue destruction.

Discussion:

Simple partial thickness burns will do well with nothing more than cleansing, debridement, and a sterile dressing. All other therapy, therefore, should be directed at making the patient more comfortable. The Silvadene cream is not always necessary, but it is soothing and may reduce the risk of infection. When it is possible to leave vesicles intact, the patient will have a shorter period of disability and will require fewer dressing changes and followup visits. If the wound must be debrided, the closed dressing technique may be more convenient and less of a mess than the open technique of washings and cream applications.

Some physicians believe it is important to remove all traces of tar from a burn. Removal can be accomplished relatively easily by using a petroleum- or petrolatum-base antibiotic ointment such as Bacitracin which will dissolve the tar. Others have found the citrus and petroleum distillate industrial cleanser, De-Solv-it, very effective as well as nontoxic, nonirritating, and odorless.

Frostbite and Frostnip

Presentation:

Frostnip occurs when skin surfaces such as the tip of the nose and ears are exposed to an environment cold enough to freeze the epidermis. These prominent exposed surfaces become blanched and develop paresthesia and numbness. As they are rewarmed, they become erythematous and at times painful.

Superficial frostbite can be either a partial or full thickness freezing of the dermis. The frozen surfaces appear white and feel soft and doughy. With rewarming these areas will become erythematous and edematous with severe pain. Blistering will occur within 24–48 hours with deeper partial thickness frostbite.

What to do:

- When there is no longer any danger of re-exposure, rapidly warm the affected part with heated blankets (warm hands in the case of frostnip) or in a warm bath (38–40°C).
- A strong analgesic such as meperidine (Demerol) or morphine may be required to control pain.
- When blistering occurs, bullae should not be ruptured. If the blisters are open, though, they should be debrided and gently cleansed with povidone-iodine and normal saline. Silvadene cream may be applied, followed by a sterile absorbent dressing.
- Patients should be provided with followup care and warned that healing of the deeper injuries may be slow and produce skin that remains very sensitive for weeks. In addition, there may be permanent damage to fingernails, long term paresthesia, and permanent cold sensitivity.

What not to do:

- Do not warm the injured skin surface while in the field if there is a chance that re-freezing will occur. Re-exposing even mildly frostbitten tissue to the cold without complete re-warming can result in additional damage.
- Do not rub the injured skin surface in an attempt to warm it. This can also create further tissue destruction.
- Do not allow the patient to smoke. Smoking causes vasoconstriction and may further decrease blood flow to the frostbitten extremity.
- Do not confuse frostnip and superficial frostbite with deep frostbite. Severe frostbite, when the deep tissue or extremity is frozen with a woody feeling and lifeless appearance, requires inpatient management and could be associated with life-threatening hypothermia.

Discussion:

Frostbite is more common in persons exposed to cold at high altitudes. The areas of the body most likely to suffer frostbite are those farthest from the trunk or large muscles: ear lobes, nose, cheeks, hands, and feet. Touching cold metal with bare hands can cause immediate frostbite, as can the spilling of gasoline or other volatile liquids on the skin at very low temperatures.

Of course, prevention is the best "treatment" for frostbite. Heavily insulated, waterproof clothing gives the best frostbite protection.

Hymenoptera (Bee/Wasp) Stings

Presentation:

Sometimes a patient comes to a hospital emergency department immediately after a painful sting because he is alarmed at the intensity of the pain or worried about developing a serious life-threatening reaction. Sometimes he seeks help the next day because of swelling, redness, and itching. Parents may not be aware that their child was stung by a bee and be concerned only about the local swelling. Erythema soon after the sting, with varying degrees of localized edema, develops. Often there is a central punctate discoloration at the site of the sting, or, rarely, a stinger may be protruding. A delayed hypersensitivity reaction will produce varying degrees of edema which can be quite dramatic when present on the face. Tenderness and, occasionally, ascending lymphangitis can occur.

What to do:

- Scrape away the stinger with the back edge of a scalpel blade or a long fingernail.
- Examine the patient for any signs of an immediate, systemic, allergic reaction (anaphylaxis), such as decreased blood pressure, generalized urticaria or erythema, or wheezing.
- Apply a cold pack to an acute sting to give pain relief and reduce swelling.
- Observe the patient with an acute sting for approximately an hour to watch for the rare occurrence of anaphylaxis.

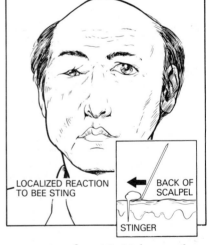

LOCALIZED REACTION TO BEE STING

BACK OF SCALPEL

STINGER

- Reassure the patient who has come in after 12–24 hours that anaphylaxis is no longer a problem.
- Prescribe hydroxyzine (Atarax) 50mg qid for itching.
- If an ascending lymphangitis is present, treat the patient with an appropriate antibiotic for 10 days (e.g., cephadryl (Duricef) 1gm qd, erythromycin 500mg qid, dicloxacillin 500mg qid).
- If an extremity is involved, have the patient keep it elevated and instruct him that the swelling may worsen if the hand or foot is held in a dependent position. This swelling may continue for

several days. Severe hand swelling may be prevented or reduced by placing the patient in a cock up splint and compression dressing. Promptly remove any rings in cases of hand stings (see p 209).

What not to do:

- Do not belittle the patient's complaint or make him feel guilty about his visit.
- Do not send the patient with an acute sting out of the ED less than one hour after the sting.
- Do not apply heat, even if an infection is suspected—the swelling and discomfort will worsen.

Discussion:

Bee stings are very painful and frightening. There are many misconceptions about the danger of bee stings, and many patients have been instructed unnecessarily to report to an ED immediately after being stung. Many of these people have only suffered localized hypersensitivity reactions in the past and are not at a significantly greater risk than the general public for developing anaphylaxis. Besides the immediate relief of pain for the acute sting, we have little more than reassurance to offer these patients. An attitude of concern and compassion along with an adequate history and physical exam will suffice in providing this reassurance.

Although it is most prudent to treat an ascending lymphangitis with an antibiotic, it should be realized that after a bee sting the resultant local cellulitis and lymphangitis is usually a chemically mediated inflammatory reaction.

Histamine is one of many components of hymenoptera venom: antihistamines may benefit the sting victim.

Superficial Sliver

Presentation:

The patient has caught himself on a sharp splinter (usually wooden) and either cannot grasp it, has broken it trying to remove it, or has found it is too large and painful to remove.

You should find a puncture wound with a tightly embedded sliver that may or may not be palpable over its entire length.

What to do:

- Locally infiltrate with 1% Xylocaine with epinephrine (no epinephrine in a digit).
- Prep with povidone-iodine and with a #15 blade, cut down over the entire length of the sliver, completely exposing it.
- The sliver can now be easily lifted out and removed.
- Cleanse the track with normal saline on a gauze sponge.
- Close the wound with sutures or wound closure strips.
- Give tetanus prophylaxis, if necessary.
- Warn the patient about the signs of infection.

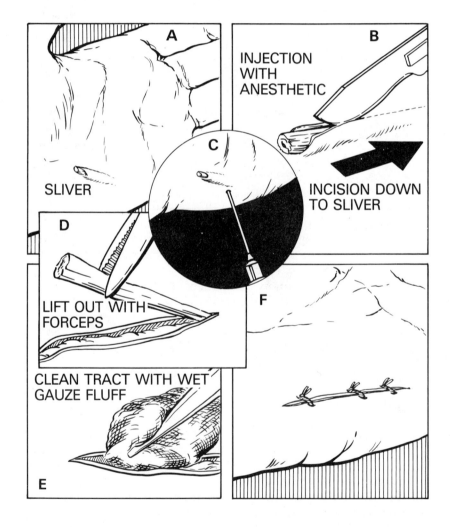

What not to do:

- Do not try to pull the sliver out.
- Do not make an incision across a neurovascular bundle, tendon, or other important structure.

Discussion:

An organic foreign body is almost certain to create an inflammatory response and become infected if any part of it is left beneath the skin. It is for this reason, along with the fact that wooden slivers tend to be friable and may break apart during removal, that complete exposure is generally necessary before the sliver can be taken out. Of course, very small and superficial slivers can be removed by loosening them and picking them out with a #18 gauge needle, avoiding the more elaborate technique described above.

If the foreign body cannot be located, explain to the patient that you do not want to do any harm by exploring and excising any further, and that therefore, you will let the splinter become infected so it will "fester" and form a "pus pocket," when it can be more easily removed. If this procedure is followed, it should always be coordinated with a followup surgeon. The patient should be placed on an antibiotic and provided with followup care within 48 hours.

When making an incision over a foreign body, always take the underlying anatomical structures into consideration. Never make an incision if there is any chance that you may sever a neurovascular bundle, tendon, or other important structure.

Pencil Point Puncture

Presentation:

The patient will tell you that he was stabbed or stuck with a sharp pencil point. He may be overtly or unconsciously worried about lead poisoning.

A small puncture wound lined with graphite tattooing will be present. The pencil tip may or may not be present, visible, or palpable. If the puncture wound is palpated, an underlying pencil point may give the patient a foreign body sensation.

What to do:

- Always reassure patient or parent that with graphite there is no danger of lead poisoning.
- Palpate and inspect for a foreign body. If uncertain, get an x ray or xerogram to rule out the presence of a foreign body (or anesthesize and explore the wound).
- Scrub wound.
- Administer tetanus prophylaxis, if necessary.
- Warn the patient or family about signs of infection, and inform them that there will be a permanent black tattoo that can be removed later if the resulting mark is cosmetically unacceptable.

What not to do:

- Do not excise the entire wound on the initial visit.

Discussion:

In order to reduce the amount of tattooing, the wound may be anesthetized and scraped (dermabraded) with the tip of a scalpel blade. It is unwise to excise the entire wound because the resultant scar might be more unsightly than the tattoo.

If a superficial pencil-tip foreign body exists, then see p 247 for an easy removal technique.

Deep punctures and/or foreign bodies may require exploratory surgery in the operating room.

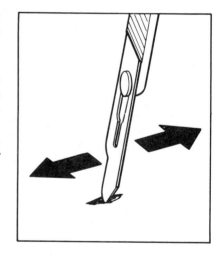

Metallic Foreign Body

Presentation:

Small, moderate-velocity metal fragments can be released when a hammer strikes a second piece of metal, such as a chisel. The patient has noticed a stinging sensation and a small puncture wound or bleeding site, and is worried that there might be something inside. B.B. shot will produce a more obvious but very similar problem. Physical findings may show an underlying, sometimes palpable, foreign body.

What to do:

- X ray the wound to document the presence and location of the suspected foreign body.
- Explain how difficult it often is to remove a small metal fleck, and that often these are left in without any problem (like shrapnel injuries).
- Inform the patient that, since it is best to remove the foreign body, you will attempt a simple technique, but that in order to avoid more damage, you will not extend your search beyond 15 minutes.
- If the foreign body is in an extremity, then it is preferable, but not essential, to establish a bloodless field (see p 225).
- Anesthetize the area with a small infiltration of 1% Xylocaine with epinephrine (avoid tissue swelling; do not use epinephrine on digits).
- Take a *blunt* stiff metal probe (not a needle) and gently slide it down the apparent track of the puncture wound. Move the probe back and forth, fanning it in all directions, until a clicking contact between the probe and the foreign body can be felt and heard. This should be repeated several times until it is certain that contact is being made with the foreign body.
- After contact is made, fix the probe in place by resting the hand holding the probe against a firm surface and then, with your other hand, cut down along the probe with a #15 scalpel blade until you reach the foreign body. Do not remove the probe.
- Reach into the incision with a pair of forceps and remove the foreign body (located at the end of the probe).
- Close the wound with strip closures or sutures.
- If the track is relatively long and the foreign body is very superficial and easily palpable beneath the skin, then it may be advantageous to eliminate the probe and just cut down directly over the foreign body.
- Provide tetanus prophylaxis.

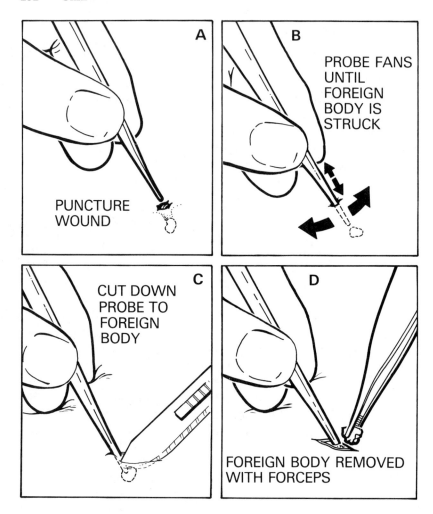

- Warn the patient about signs of developing infection.
- If you are unable to locate the foreign body in 15 minutes, inform the patient that the wound will probably heal without any problem; but, should it become infected, it can be successfully treated with an antibiotic, and the foreign body can be more easily removed if an abscess or "pus pocket" forms. In addition, these small foreign bodies may migrate to the skin surface over a period of months or years, at which time they can be more easily removed.
- Always provide the patient with a physician who can perform the necessary followup care.

What not to do:

- Do not cut down on the metal probe if there is any possibility of cutting across a neurovascular bundle, tendon or other important structure.
- Do not attempt to cut down to the foreign body, unless it is very superficial, without a probe in place and in contact with the foreign body.

Discussion:

These moderate-velocity metallic foreign bodies rarely travel deeply to the subcutaneous tissue, but you must consider a potentially serious injury when these objects strike the eye.

When you honestly inform the patient how difficult it can be to locate and remove these foreign bodies, you help to place yourself in a win/win situation. If you find the foreign body the patient now appreciates how difficult it was for you. If you don't find the foreign body the patient is impressed with the insight and knowledge you have demonstrated about the difficulty of foreign body removal. In either event, if you remove your ego from this surgical procedure you comfortably stop searching after 15 minutes.

X rays are needed in documenting the presence of a foreign body and its location relative to significant anatomic structures. X rays are usually of little value, though, in locating metallic flecks. Even when skin markers are used, because of variances in the angle of the x ray beam to the film, relative to the skin marker and foreign body, the apparent location of the foreign body is often significantly different from the real location. An incision made over the apparent location, therefore, usually produces no foreign body.

In an effort to reduce the possibility of a malpractice suit, it is advisable to inform the patient if you are going to leave the foreign body beneath the skin. Give the patient realistic expectations as to the possibility of complications. Many emergency physicians would consult with a surgeon before sending a patient out with an embedded foreign body.

Tick Removal

Presentation:

The patient arrives with a tick attached to the skin, most often the scalp, usually frightened or disgusted and is almost always concerned about developing "tick fever."

What to do:

- Promptly remove the tick. Grasp the tick with a pair of forceps and slowly pull up until the tick mouth parts separate from the skin.
- If the mouth parts remain embedded, anesthetize the area with an infiltration of 1% Xylocaine and use a #10 scalpel blade to scrape (dermabrade) these fragments away.

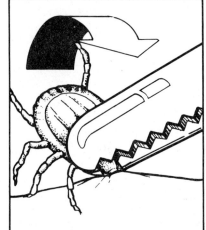

- If the mouth parts still remain embedded, it will be necessary to make an eliptical excision of the area and suture it closed.
- Instruct the patient or family to record the patient's temperature twice a day for the next 2 weeks and to notify a physician or return to the ED at the first sign of a temperature above the baseline.
- Reassure the patient and family that the likelihood of developing Rocky Mountain spotted fever is very small (1%) and that if it should occur, prompt treatment will be quite effective upon development of fever.

What not to do:

- Do not spend a lot of time or effort attempting to use heat, occlusion, or caustics to remove a tick. A multitude of techniques have been promoted, but they may increase the chance of infection by making the tick regurgitate.
- Do not contaminate your fingers with potentially infected tick products.
- Do not administer prophylactic antibiotic therapy. The treatment is not only in all likelihood unnecessary, but, in the event the patient is infected, it may interfere with the initiation of the patient's immune response. Withhold antibiotics until symptoms occur.

Discussion:

Ixodes dammini, the tiny deer tick of New England, carries babesiosis and Lyme disease. *Dermacentor variabilis*, the dog tick, is the major vector of Rocky Mountain spotted fever, which is also carried by *D. andersoni*, the western wood tick, and *Amblyomma americanum*, the lone star tick. *A. americanum* has particularly long

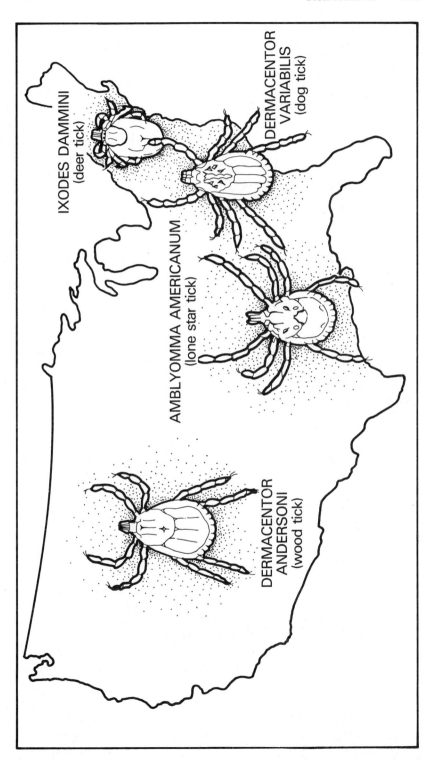

mouth parts, and is most likely to require the dissection described above (its larvae are also capable of infesting human hosts).

Other diseases carried by ticks include tick paralysis (usually cured by removing the tick), Colorado tick fever, relapsing fever, Q fever, and tularemia.

Cutaneous Abscess/Pustule

Presentation:

With or without a history of minor trauma (such as an embedded foreign body) the patient has localized pain, swelling and redness of the skin. The area is warm, firm, and, usually, fluctuant to palpation. There is sometimes surrounding cellulitis or lymphangitis and, in the more serious case, fever.

A pustule will appear only as a cloudy tender vesicle surrounded by some redness and induration, and occasionally will be the source of an ascending lymphangitis.

What to do:

- A pustule does not require any anesthesia for drainage. Simply snip open the cutaneous roof with fine scissors or an inverted #11 blade, grasp an edge with pickups and excise the entire overlying surface. Cleanse the open surface with normal saline and cover it with povidone-iodine ointment and a dressing.
- When the location of an abscess cavity is uncertain, attempt to aspirate it with a #18 gauge needle after prepping the area with povidone-iodine. If an abscess cavity cannot be located, send the patient out on antibiotics and intermittent warm moist compresses and have him seen again in 24 hours.
- When the abscess is pointing or has been located by needle aspiration, prepare the overlying skin for incision and drainage with povidone-iodine solution. Anesthetize the area with a regional field block, accomplished by injecting a ring of subcutaneous 1% lidocaine solution approximately 1cm away from the erythematous border of the abscess. In addition, inject lidocaine into the roof of the abscess along the line of the projected incision.
- The incision should be made with a #15 blade at the most dependent area of fluctuance. It should be large and directed along the relaxed skin tension lines to reduce future scarring.

- In larger abscesses insert a hemostat into the cavity to break up any loculated collections of pus. The cavity may then be irrigated with normal saline and loosely packed with Iodoform or plain gauze. Leave a small wick of this gauze protruding through the incision to allow for continued drainage and easy removal after 48 hours.
- The patient should be instructed to use intermittent warm water soaks or compresses for a few days when there is no packing used or after packing is removed.
- A dressing should be provided to collect continued drainage.

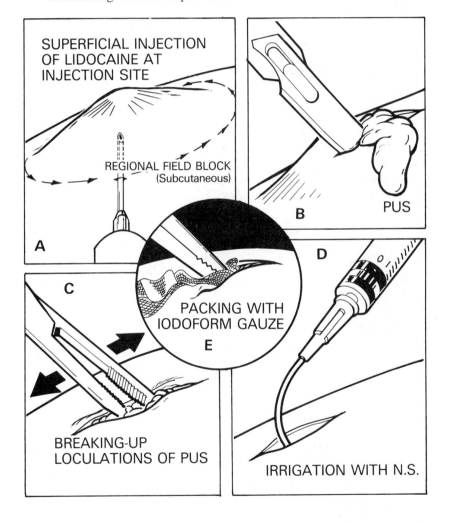

SUPERFICIAL INJECTION OF LIDOCAINE AT INJECTION SITE

REGIONAL FIELD BLOCK (Subcutaneous)

A

B

PUS

C

D

PACKING WITH IODOFORM GAUZE

E

BREAKING-UP LOCULATIONS OF PUS

IRRIGATION WITH N.S.

What not to do:

- Do not incise an abscess that lies in close proximity to a major vessel, such as in the axilla, groin or antecubital space, without first confirming its location and nature by needle aspiration. An incision into a mycotic aneurysm could result in profound hemorrhage.

- Do not treat deep infections of the hands as simple cutaneous abscesses. When significant pain and swelling exists, or there is pain or range of motion of a finger, seek surgical consultation.

Discussion:

Either trauma or obstruction of the eccrine or exocrine glands in the skin can lead to cutaneous abscesses. Incision and drainage is the definitive therapy for these lesions and, therefore, routine cultures and antibiotics are generally not indicated. Exceptions exist in the immunologically suppressed patient, the toxic, febrile patient, or where there is a large area of cellulitis or lymphangitis, in which cases an antibiotic can be selected on the basis of a Gram stain or presumptively based on body location.

It is sometimes not possible to achieve total regional anesthesia for incision and drainage of an abscess, perhaps because local tissue acidosis neutralizes local anesthetics. In such cases, additional analgesia may be obtained by premedication with narcotics or brief inhalation of nitrous oxide.

Erysipelas/Cellulitis/Lymphangitis

Presentation:

The cardinal signs of infection (pain, redness, warmth, and swelling) are present. *Erysipelas* is very superficial and bright red with indurated, sharply demarcated borders. *Cellulitis* is deeper, involves the subcutaneous tissue, and has an indistinct advancing border. *Lymphangitis* has minimal induration and an unmistakable linear pattern ascending along lymphatic channels.

These superficial skin infections are often preceded by minor trauma or the presence of a foreign body, and are most common in patients who have predisposing factors such as diabetes, arterial or venous insufficiency, and lymphatic drainage obstruction. They may be associated with an abscess or they may have no clear-cut origin.

With any of these skin infections the patient may have tender lymphadenopathy proximal to the site of infection and may or may not have signs of systemic toxicity (fever, rigors, and listlessness).

What to do:

- Look for a possible source of infection and remove it. Debride and cleanse any wound, remove any foreign body or drain any abscess.
- When the patient is very toxic, or if discoloration of the affected extremity is present, get medical consultation and prepare for hospitalization. Obtain a CBC and blood cultures and get x rays to look for gas-forming organisms. Hospitalization should also be strongly considered when deep facial cellulitis is present or the patient has a deep infection of the hand.
- If there is low-grade fever, or none at all, you can usually treat on an outpatient basis. Prescribe dicloxacillin 500mg qid × 10d, erythromycin 500mg qid × 10d or cefadroxil (Duricef) 1gm qd × 10d. Instruct the patient to keep the infected part at rest and elevated and to use intermittent warm moist compresses.
- Followup within 24–48 hours to insure that the therapy has been adequate. Infections still worsening after 48 hours of outpatient treatment may require hospital admission for better immobilization, elevation, and intravenous antibiotics.

Discussion:

The most common etiologic agents are Group A β-hemolytic strep or *Staphylococcus aureus*. Erysipelas and lymphangitis are usually a result of Group A β-hemolytic strep alone although *S. aureus* may produce a similar picture. *H. influenzae* must be strongly considered as the etiologic agent in the toxic child with a markedly elevated white blood cell count or facial cellulitis.

It may be easier to evaluate on followup whether a cellulitis is improving or not if the initial margin of redness, swelling, tenderness, or warmth was marked on the skin with a ball point pen. Because response to treatment is often equivocal at 24 hours, re-evaluation is usually best scheduled at 48 hours.

Pyogenic Granuloma (Proud Flesh)

Presentation:

Often there is a history of a laceration several days to a few weeks before presentation in the ED. The wound has not healed and now bleeds with every slight trauma.

Objective findings usually include a crusted, sometimes purulent, collection of friable granulation tissue arising from a moist, sometimes hemorrhagic wound. There are usually no signs of a deep tissue infection.

What to do:

- Cleanse the area with hydrogen peroxide and Betadine.
- Cauterize the granulation tissue with a silver nitrate stick until it is completely discolored.
- Dress the wound after applying Betadine ointment and have the patient repeat ointment and dressings 2–3 times per day until healed.
- Warn the patient about the potential signs of developing infection.

What not to do:

- Do not cauterize any lesion that by history and appearance might be neoplastic in nature. These lesions should be referred for complete excision and pathologic examination.
- Do not cauterize a large or extensive lesion. These should also be completely excised.

Discussion:

It is not uncommon for a secondary cellulitis to develop after cauterizing the granuloma. It is therefore reasonable to place a patient on a short course (3–4 days) of a high dose (500mg qid) antibiotic (e.g., dicloxacillin, cephalexin, erythromycin) when the wound is located on a distal extremity.

Zipper—Caught on Penis or Chin

Presentation:

Usually a child has gotten dressed too quickly and accidentally pulled up skin in his zipper. The skin becomes entrapped and crushed between the teeth and the slide of the zipper, thereby painfully attaching the article of clothing to the body part involved (most often the penis or the area beneath the chin).

What to do:

- Paint the area with a small amount of povidone-iodine and infiltrate the skin with 1% lidocaine (plain). This will allow the comfortable manipulation of the zipper and the article of clothing.
- Cut the zipper away from the article of clothing to leave yourself with a less cumbersome problem.
- Cut the slide of the zipper in half with a pair of metal snips or an orthopedic pin cutter. The patient is less likely to be frightened if this procedure is kept hidden from his view.
- Pull the exposed zipper teeth apart, cleanse the crushed skin, and apply an ointment such as povidone-iodine.
- Tetanus prophylaxis should be administered as needed.

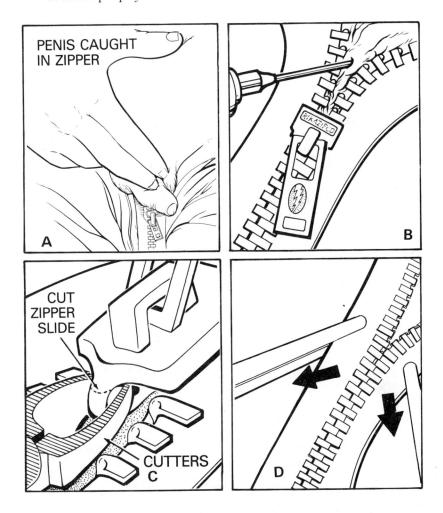

What not to do:

- Do not destroy the entire article of clothing by cutting into it. You only need to cut the zipper away allowing repair of the clothing.
- Do not excise an area of skin or perform a circumcision; it only creates unnecessary morbidity for the patient.

Discussion:

Newer plastic zippers have made this problem less common than in the past, but it still occurs, and it is a very grateful patient who is released from this entrapment.

Contusions (Bruises)

Presentation:

The patient has fallen or been struck at a site where now there is point tenderness, swelling, ecchymosis, hematoma, or pain with use. On physical examination, there is no loss of function of muscles and tendons (beyond mild splinting because of pain), no instability of bones and ligaments, and no crepitus or tenderness produced by remote stress (such as weight-bearing on the leg or manual flexing of a rib).

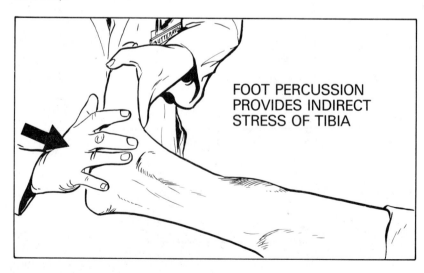

FOOT PERCUSSION
PROVIDES INDIRECT
STRESS OF TIBIA

What to do:

- Take a thorough history to ascertain the mechanism of injury and perform a complete examination to document structural integrity and intact function.
- Reserve x rays for possible foreign bodies and bony injury, suggested by point tenderness on indirect percussion or stressing of bone. The yield is very low when x rays are ordered on the basis of pain or swelling.
- Explain to the patient that swelling will peak in 1–3 days, but that swelling and resultant stiffness and pain may be reduced by good treatment during the first 1–2 days. Prescribe:
  a) resting the affected part,
  b) immobilization (the ultimate in rest, best achieved with a splint),
  c) elevation of the affected part (ideally, above the level of the heart), and
  d) cold (usually an ice bag, wrapped in a damp towel, applied to the injury for 10–20 minutes per hour).
- Explain to the patient the late migration and color change of ecchymoses, so that green or purple discoloration appearing farther down the limb a week after the injury does not frighten him into thinking he has another injury.
- Arrange for re-evaluation and followup.

What not to do:

- Do not apply an elastic bandage to the middle of a limb, where it may act as a tourniquet. Include all of the distal limb in the wrapping.
- Do not confuse patients with instructions for application of heat and exercises to prevent stiffness and atrophy. Concentrate on the here-and-now therapy of the acute injury; namely, rest, immobilization, elevation, and cold—all designed to decrease acute edema. Leave other instructions to followup and physical therapy consultants. Patients who confuse today's correct therapy with next week's can complicate their problem.
- Do not take for granted that all of your patients understand rest, immobilization, elevation, and cold. Walking on a fresh foot injury or soaking it for long periods in ice water or Epsom salts are not usually therapeutic.

Discussion:

The acute therapy of contusions concentrates upon reduction of the acute edema, and all other components of treatment are postponed for 3–4 days, until the edema is reduced. Patients need to know this time course, and must understand that the more the edema can be reduced, the sooner injuries can heal, function return, and pain decrease. Edema of hands and feet is especially slow to resolve, because these structures usually hang in a dependent position, and require much modification of activity to rest.

Urticaria (Hives)

Presentation:

The patient is generally very uncomfortable, with intense itching. There may be a history of similar episodes and perhaps a known precipitating agent (bee sting, food, or drug). Most commonly the patient will only have a rash. Sometimes this is accompanied by edematous swelling of the lips, face and/or hands (angioedema). In the more severe cases, patients may have wheezing, laryngeal edema and/or frank cardiovascular collapse (anaphylaxis).

The urticarial rash consists of sharply defined, slightly raised wheals surrounded by erythema and tending to be circular or serpiginous. Each eruption is transient, lasting no more than 8–12 hours, but it may be replaced by new lesions in different locations.

What to do:

- Attempt to elicit a precipitating cause, including drugs, foods, stress, or an underlying infection or illness (e.g., collagen vascular disease, malignancy, or, when accompanied by arthralgias, anicteric hepatitis).
- For immediate relief of severe pruritis, administer 0.3cc of epinephrine (1:1000) subcutaneously.
- For continued relief administer hydroxyzine (Vistaril) 50mg im or po.
- For prolonged relief prescribe hydroxyzine (Atarax) 25–50mg or cyproheptadine hydrochloride (Periactin) 4mg q6h for the next 48 hours. For the more severe cases, it may also be helpful to add ephedrine 25mg q6h to the therapy.
- Inform the patient that the cause of hives cannot be determined in the vast majority of cases. Let him know that the condition is usually of minor consequence but can at times become chronic, and, under unusual circumstances, is associated with other illnesses. Therefore, the patient should be provided with elective followup care.

What not to do:

- Do not allow the patient to take aspirin. Many patients experience a worsening of their symptoms with the use of aspirin. Morphine, codeine, reserpine, and alcohol, as well as certain food additives such as tartrazine dye, are often allergens or potentiate allergic reactions, and benzoates should probably also be avoided.
- Do not use systemic steroids unless all other therapeutic methods have failed.

Discussion:

Although the treatment of anaphylactic shock is beyond the scope of this book, when hypotension is present, aggressive intravenous fluid therapy should be instituted, along with the intramuscular or intravenous administration of epinephrine.

Simple urticaria affects approximately 20% of the population at some time. This local reaction is due at least in part to the release of histamines and other vasoactive peptides from mast cells following an IgE mediated antigen-antibody reaction. This results in vasodilatation and increased vascular permeability, with the leaking of protein and fluid into extravascular spaces.

The heavier concentration of mast cells within the lips, face, and hands explains why these areas are more commonly affected. In asthma, the bronchial tree is more affected, whereas with eczema, the skin in knee and elbow creases is most heavily invested with mast cells and the first to develop hives.

Pityriasis Rosea

Presentation:

Patients with this benign disorder often seek acute medical help because of the worrisome sudden spread of a rash that began with one local skin lesion. This "herald patch" may develop anywhere on the body and appears as a round 2–6cm mildly erythematous scaling plaque. There is no change for a period of several days to two weeks; then the rash appears, composed of small (1–2cm), pale, salmon-colored, oval macules or plaques with a coarse surface surrounded by a rim of fine scales. The distribution is truncal with the long axis of the oval lesions running in the planes of cleavage of the skin (parallel to the ribs). The condition may be asymptomatic or accompanied by varying degrees of pruritis and, occasionally, mild malaise. The lesions will gradually extend in size and may become confluent with one another. The rash persists for 6–8 weeks, then completely disappears. Recurrences are uncommon.

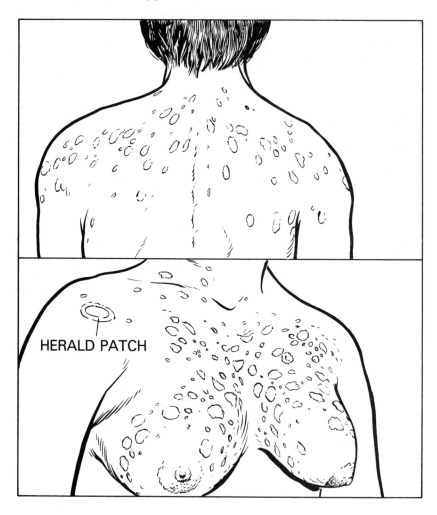

HERALD PATCH

What to do:

- Reassure the patient about the benign nature of this disease. Be sympathetic and let him know that you understand how frightening it can seem.
- Draw blood for serologic testing for syphilis (e.g., VDRL). Secondary syphilis can mimic pityriasis rosea. Make a note to track down the results of the test.

- Provide relief from pruritis by prescribing hydroxyzine (Atarax) 50mg q6h or an emollient such as Lubriderm. Tepid corn starch baths (1 cup in ½ tub of water) may also be comforting. Exposure to tanning doses of sunlight or sunlamp will reduce itching and shorten the duration of the rash.
- Inform the patient that he should anticipate a 6–8 week course of the disease, but to seek followup care if the rash does not resolve within 12 weeks.

What not to do:

- Do not leave the patient with a sense of guilt for having sought emergency care. Nobody really benefits from this, and in fact, the patient may turn out to have a serious condition, such as secondary syphilis.
- Do not use topical or systemic steroids. These are only effective in the most severe inflammatory varieties of this syndrome.
- Do not send off a serologic test for syphilis without assuring the results will be seen and acted upon.

Discussion:

Pityriasis rosea is seen most commonly in adolescents and young adults during the spring and fall seasons. It may be viral in origin but the true etiology is uncertain. The "herald patch" may not be seen in 20–30% of the cases and there are many variations from the classic presentation described. Other diagnostic considerations besides syphilis include tinea corporis, seborrheic dermatitis, acute psoriasis, and tinea versicolor.

Tinea (Athlete's Foot, ringworm)

Presentation:

Patients usually seek emergency care for "athlete's foot," "jock itch," or "ringworm" when pruritis is severe or when secondary infection causes pain and swelling. Tinea pedis is usually seen as interdigital scaling, maceration, and fissuring. At times tense vesicular lesions will be present instead. Tinea cruris is usually a moist, mildly erythematous eruption symmetrically affecting both groin and upper inner thigh. Tinea corporis appears (most often on the hairless skin of children) as dry erythematous lesions with sharp annular and arciform borders that are scaling or vesicular.

What to do:

- When microscopic examination of skin scrapings is readily available, definite identification of the lesion can be made by looking for the presence of hyphae or spores (resembling microscopic spaghetti and meatballs) in the scabs or hair. Treatment can be started presumptively when microscopic examination is not easily accomplished.
- With signs of secondary infection, begin treatment first with wet compresses of Burow's solution (2 pks of Domeboro powder in 1 pint water) ½ hr every 3–4 hours. With signs of deep infection (cellulitis, lymphangitis) begin systemic antibiotics in addition [cefadroxil (Duricef)] 1gm qd × 5–7 day or dicloxacillin 250–500mg qid × 5–7 days).
- With inflammation and weeping lesions, a topical antifungal and steroid cream such as (Vioform-Hydrocortisone) in addition to the compresses will be most effective. Warn patients that this medication will stain white clothing yellow.
- Alternative topical therapy can be prescribed. Clotrimazole (Lotrimin), miconazole (Micatin) haloprogin (Halotex) and tolnaftate (Tinactin) solution or cream applied tid will cause involution of most superficial lesions within 1–3 weeks.

What not to do:

- Do not attempt to treat deep, painful fungal infections of the scalp (tinea capitis) with local therapy. A deep boggy swelling (tinea kerion) or patchy hair loss with inflammation and scaling requires systemic antifungal antibiotics (e.g., griseofulvin).
- Do not treat with corticosteroids alone. They will reduce signs and symptoms, but allow increased fungal growth.

Discussion:

Tinea versicolor, except for its somewhat unsightly appearance, is asymptomatic. Its presentation to an acute care facility usually is incidental with some other problem. There is, however, no reason to ignore this fungal infection, which causes cosmetically unpleasant, irregular patches of varying pigmentation that tend to be lighter than the surrounding skin in the summer and darker than the surrounding skin in the winter. Simply prescribe a 25% sodium hyposulfite lotion (Tinver) bid for several weeks. Superficial scaling will resolve in a few days and the pigmentary changes will slowly clear over a period of several months.

Herpes Zoster (Shingles)

Presentation:

Patients complain of pain, paresthesia, or an itch that covers a specific dermatome and then develops into a characteristic rash. Prior to the onset of the rash, zoster can be confused with pleuritic or cardiac pain, cholecystitis, or ureteral colic. Approximately 3–5 days from the onset of symptoms, an eruption of erythematous macules and papules will appear, first posteriorly then spreading anteriorly along the course of the involved nerve segment. In most instances grouped vesicles will appear within the next 24 hrs. Herpes zoster most often occurs in the thoracic and cervical segments.

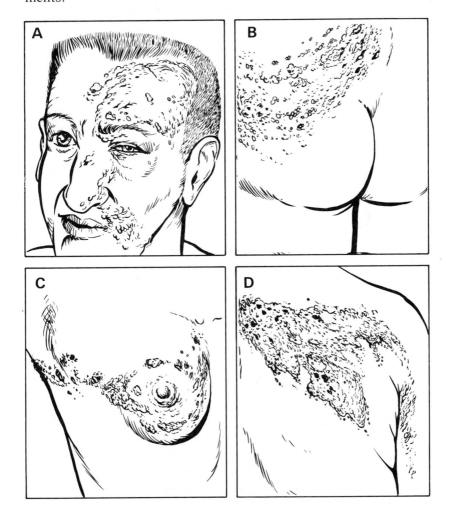

What to do:

- Prescribe analgesics appropriate for the level of pain the patient is experiencing. Anti-inflammatory medications may help, but narcotics are often required (e.g., Percocet q4h).
- Cool compresses with Burow's solution will be comforting (e.g., Domeboro powder, 2 pkts in 1 pint of water).
- Dressing the lesions with gauze and splinting them with an elastic wrap may also help bring relief.
- Secondary infection should be treated with povidone-iodine (Betadine) ointment.
- In patients over 60 years of age, systemic steroids should be prescribed at the onset to decrease the incidence of postherpetic neuralgia. Prednisone 60mg qd × 7d should be administered, followed by 30mg qd for another 7 days then 15mg qd for the final 7 days. This treatment will be of no value if started after 7 days from the onset of the eruption.
- Ocular lesions should be evaluated by an ophthalmologist and treated with topical ophthalmic corticosteroids. Although topical steroids are contraindicated in herpes simplex keratitis, because they allow deeper corneal injury, this does not appear to be a problem with herpes zoster ophthalmicus.

What not to do:

- Do not prescribe systemic steroids for patients at high risk, i.e., with latent tuberculosis, peptic ulcer, diabetes mellitus, hypertension, and congestive heart failure.

Discussion:

Zoster results from reactivation of latent herpes varicella/zoster (chickenpox) virus residing in dorsal root or cranial nerve ganglion cells. Two-thirds of the patients are over 40 years old. This is a self-limiting, localized disease and usually heals within 3–4 weeks. Postherpetic neuralgia in patients over 60 years old, however, can be an extremely painful, recurrent misery, and deserves prophylaxis when possible.

Pediculosis (Lice, crabs)

Presentation:

Patients arrive with emotions ranging from annoyance to sheer disgust at the discovery of an infestation with lice or crabs and request acute medical care. There may be extreme pruritis and the patient may bring in a sample of the creature to show you. The adult forms of head lice can be very difficult to find but their oval, light gray eggs (nits) can be readily found firmly attached to the hairs above the ears and toward the occiput. Secondary impetigo and furunculosis can occur. The adult forms of pubic lice (crabs) are more easily found, but their light yellow gray color still makes them difficult to see. Small black dots present in infested areas represent either ingested blood in adult lice or their excreta.

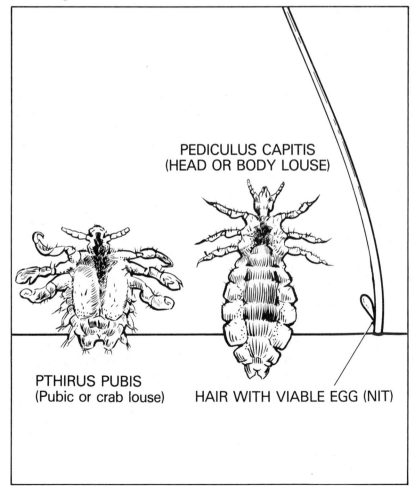

PEDICULUS CAPITIS
(HEAD OR BODY LOUSE)

PTHIRUS PUBIS
(Pubic or crab louse)   HAIR WITH VIABLE EGG (NIT)

What to do:

- Instruct the patient and other close contacts on the use of pyrethrins with piperonyl butoxide (RID), an over-the-counter louse remedy which should be applied undiluted to the hair until the affected area is entirely wet. After 10 minutes the infested area should be shampooed and thoroughly rinsed with warm water. This treatment may be repeated if necessary, but it should not be used more than twice within a 24 hr period and it is advisable to wait a week before repeating treatment should reinfestation occur.
- Families should also be instructed to disinfect sheets and clothing by machine washing in hot water, machine drying on the hot cycle for 20 minutes, ironing, dry cleaning, or storage in plastic bags for two weeks. Combs and brushes should be soaked in 2% Lysol or heated in water to about 65°C for 10 minutes.
- Application of a 1:1 solution of white vinegar and water may help to loosen nits prior to removal with a fine-toothed comb.

What not to do:

- Do not have the family use commercial sprays (R&C Spray III or Li-Ban Spray) to control lice on inanimate objects. Their use is no more effective than vacuuming.
- Do not let patients use lindane (Kwell) shampoo on mucous membranes, around the eyes, on acutely inflamed areas, and do not prescribe it for pregnant women and infants. It is absorbed and can be toxic to the central nervous system.

Discussion:

Head and pubic lice are obligatory bloodsucking ectoparasites whose eggs are firmly attached to the hair shafts near the skin, and incubate for about a week before hatching. Nits located more than one-half inch from the scalp are no longer viable.

A common alternate treatment for lice is the use of lindane shampoo which is only available by prescription. One ounce is worked into the affected area for four minutes and then thoroughly rinsed out. Because of the very toxic nature of lindane, its use should be reserved for those cases that fail to respond to pyrethrins (RID). Treatment with either substance may not be ovicidal and therefore re-treatment after 7 to 10 days is often recommended.

Scabies

Presentation:

Patients will rush to the emergency department shortly after having gone to bed, unable to sleep because of severe itching. Papules and vesicles (marking deposition of eggs) along thread-like tracks (mite burrows) are chiefly found in the interdigital web spaces as well as on the volar aspects of the wrists, antecubital fossa, olecranon area, nipples, umbilicus, lower abdomen, genitalia and gluteal cleft. Secondary bacterial infection is often present.

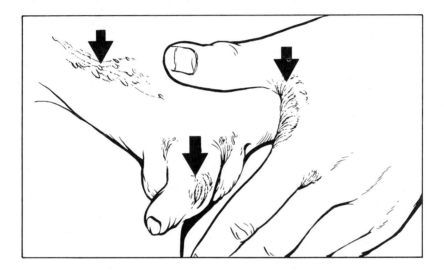

What to do:

- Attempt identification of the mite by placing mineral oil over the papule or vesicle at the proximal end of a track and scraping it with a #15 scalpel blade onto a microscope slide. Examine it under low magnification for either the mite or its oval eggs or fecal concretions.
- If the clinical picture is convincing, treatment should be instituted without the help of microscopic examination and even in the face of negative scrapings.
- Treat with lindane (Kwell) lotion to the entire body from the neck down. Concentrate on the affected areas. The patient should apply this prescription medication and leave it on for 24 hours before washing it off (60–120ml is required for the average adult). It may be necessary to repeat this treatment after 1 week, but not sooner. Tell the patient that the itching will not

go away at once, but that this does not mean the Kwell was ineffective. Dead mites and eggs continue to itch as they are absorbed by the body.

- Clothing, bedding, and towels should be washed with hot water or dry cleaned to prevent reinfection.
- An antipruritic agent such as hydroxyzine (Atarax) 25mg q6h can be prescribed for comfort.

What not to do:

- Do not use Kwell on infants, young children, or pregnant women. Up to 10% of this pesticide may be absorbed percutaneously, producing seizures or CNS toxicity, and therefore an alternative treatment should be sought. Crotamiton (Eurax) cream applied twice during a 48 hr period will be effective and also acts as an antipruritic agent.

Discussion:

Scabies is caused by infestation with the mite *Sarcoptes scabiei*. The female mite, which is just visible to the human eye, excavates a burrow in the stratum corneum and travels about 2mm a day for about 1–2 months before dying. During this time she lays eggs which reach maturity in about 3 weeks.

Scabies is transmitted principally through close personal contact, but may be transmitted through clothing, linens, or towels.

Severe pruritis is probably caused by an acquired sensitivity to the organism and is first noted 2–4 weeks after primary infestation.

Sometimes nonspecific, pruritic, generalized maculopapular excoriated rash, turns out, after a therapeutic trial of Kwell, to have been an atypical case of scabies.

Impetigo

Presentation:

Parents will usually bring their children in because they are developing unsightly skin lesions, which may be pruritic and are found most often on the face or other exposed areas. Streptococcal lesions consist of irregular or somewhat circular, red, oozing erosions, often covered with a yellow-brown crust. These may be surrounded by smaller erythematous macular or vesiculopustular areas. Staphylococcal lesions present as bullae which are quickly replaced by a thin shiny crust over an erythematous base. Impetigo is very contagious among infants and young children and may be associated with poor hygiene or predisposing skin eruptions such as chicken pox, scabies, and atopic and contact dermatitis.

What to do:

- Prescribe a 10 day course of erythromycin or penicillin VK (250mg qid), or one intramuscular injection of benzathine penicillin (600,000 units im for children 6 years and younger, 1.2 million units im for children over 7 years.) For suspected staphylococcal infections use dicloxacillin (250mg qid) in place of penicillin (or prescribe erythromycin or cefadroxil).
- Have parents soften and cleanse crusts with warm soapy compresses, preferably a povidone-iodine (Betadine) scrub two to three times per day.
- Washings should be followed by the application of a povidone-iodine (Betadine) ointment.

What not to do:

- Do not rely on topical antibiotics alone to eliminate either streptococcal or staphylococcal lesions.
- Do not routinely culture these lesions. This is only indicated for unusual lesions or lesions that fail to respond to routine therapy.

Discussion:

Impetigo is usually self-limiting and it is believed that antibiotic treatment does not alter the subsequent incidence of secondary glomerulonephritis. Systemic antibiotics are indicated, though, because they shorten the course of this unpleasant disease, decrease the number of recurrences and reduce the streptococcal carrier rate, thereby preventing further spread.

Diaper Rash

Presentation:

An infant has worn a wet diaper too long, and has developed an uncomfortable rash, which may range fron simple redness to macerated and superinfected skin. Hallmarks of Candida infection are often present, including intensely red, raw areas, satellite lesions, and white exudate.

What to do:

- Instruct the parents that it is imperative that the child go "bare" and wear no diaper until the rash has healed. This may increase the laundry load, but it allows the skin to dry, avoid physical trauma, and restore its natural defenses. This is usually all that is necessary to clear up a diaper rash in 2–3 days, but . . .
- To speed recovery from the frequent superinfection of Candida (present in the feces) and less-frequent superinfection with other dermatophytes, you may add topical treatment with clotrimazole (Lotrimin) or nystatin (mycostatin) cream, applied 3 or 4 times daily until the rash has been healed for 2 days.
- Make sure the family has a pediatrician for further followup.

What not to do:

- Do not let the parents be distracted by drying or emolient medications. Going bare is the basis of treatment.
- Do not recommend talcum powder or "talcum free" powders for use when diapers are changed. They add little in terms of medication or absorbency, and are occasionally aspirated by infants as their diapers are being changed.

Discussion:

Superinfection with Candida is common enough to treat presumptively in every case of diaper rash.

12

Prophylaxis

Tetanus Prophylaxis

Presentation:

The patient may have stepped on a nail, or sustained any sort of laceration or puncture wound, when the question of tetanus prophylaxis comes up.

What to do:

- If the patient has not had tetanus immunization in the past 5 years, give adult tetanus and diphtheria toxoid (Td) 0.5ml im.
- If there is any doubt the patient has had his original series of three tetanus immunizations, add tetanus immune globulin (e.g., Hyper-Tet) 250mg im, and make arrangements for him to complete the full series with additional immunizations at 4 to 6 weeks and 6 to 12 months.

What not to do:

- Do not assume adequate immunization. The groups most at risk in the US today are immigrants, elderly women, and rural southern blacks. Veterans usually have been immunized. Many patients incorrectly assume they were immunized during a surgical procedure. Having had tetanus does not confer immunity.
- Do not give tetanus immunizations indiscriminately. Besides being wasteful, too-frequent immunizations are more likely to cause reactions, probably of the antigen-antibody type. (Surprisingly, the routine of administering toxoid and immune globulin simultaneously in two deltoid muscles does not seem to cause mutual inactivation or serum sickness.)

- Do not believe every story of allergy to tetanus toxoid (which is actually quite rare). Is the patient actually describing a local reaction, the predictable serum sickness of horse serum, or a reaction to older, less pure preparations of toxoid? The only absolute contraindication is a history of immediate hypersensitivity—urticaria, bronchospasm, or shock. Tetanus toxoid is safe for use in pregnancy.
- Do not give pediatric tetanus and diphtheria toxoid (TD) to an adult. TD contains 8 times as much diphtheria toxoid as Td.

Discussion:

There continue to be about 100 cases of tetanus in the US each year. The CDC recommends everyone receive Td every 10 years, but somehow physicians and patients alike forget tetanus prophylaxis until after a wound. Because tetanus has followed negligible injuries, the concept of the "tetanus-prone wound" is not really helpful. The CDC recommends including a small dose of diphtheria toxin (Td) but, because this is more apt to cause local reactions, you may want to revert to plain tetanus toxoid (TT) in patients who have complained of such reactions.

Rabies Prophylaxis

Presentation:

A possibly contagious animal has bitten the patient, or the animal's saliva contaminated an abrasion or mucous membrane.

What to do:

- Clean and debride the wound thoroughly. Irrigate with soap and water or 1% benzalkonium chloride and rinse with normal saline if rabies is suspected.
- Know the local prevalence of rabies, or ask someone who knows (e.g., local health department).
- If the offending animal was an apparently healthy dog or cat, arrange to have the animal observed for ten days. During that period, an animal affected with rabies will show symptoms and should be sacrificed and examined for rabies using a fluorescent rabies antibody (FRA) technique. If the test is positive, begin prophylaxis with rabies immune globulin and human diploid

cell vaccine. If the animal is not available for observation, the decision of whether to provide rabies prophylaxis depends on the local prevalence of rabies in domestic animals, rodents, and lagomorphs.

- If a wild animal (e.g., bat, coyote, fox, opossum, raccoon, skunk) capable of transmitting rabies is caught, it should be killed and sent to the local public health department so the brain can be examined with immunofluorescence. If the animal did not appear to be healthy, or if the bite is on the patient's face, the patient should be started on RIG and HDCV in the meantime and stopped only if the test is negative.

     If the offending wild animal was not captured, no matter how normal-appearing, assume it was rabid, and give a full course of RIG and HDCV.
- Provide passive immunity with 20IU/kg of rabies immune globulin, half im and half infiltrating the area of the bite.
- Begin rapid immunization with human diploid cell vaccine, 1ml im.
- Make arrangements for repeat doses of HDCV at 3, 7, 14, and 28 days post exposure, and an antibody level following the series.

What not to do:

- Do not treat the bites of rodents and lagomorphs (hamsters, rabbits, squirrels, rats, etc.) unless rabies is endemic in your area. As of 1984, rodent and lagomorph bites have not caused human rabies in the United States.
- Do not omit rabies immune globulin. Treatment failures have resulted from giving HDCV alone.

Discussion:

The older duck embryo vaccine for rabies required 21 injections, and produced more side effects and less of an antibody response than the new human diploid cell vaccine. Sometimes, neurological symptoms would arise from DEV treatment, raising the agonizing question of whether they represented early signs of rabies or side effects of the treatment, and thus whether treatment should be continued or discontinued. It is much easier nowadays to initiate immunization with HDCV and follow through, because side effects are minimal and antibody response excellent.

The incubation period of rabies varies from weeks to months, roughly in proportion to the length of the axons up which the virus must propagate to the brain, which is why prophylaxis is especially urgent in facial bites.

Hepatitis A Prophylaxis

Presentation:

Those who may benefit include people who share eating and drinking utensils with an infectious hepatitis A patient; people who ate shellfish contaminated with hepatitis A, or people who will be traveling to endemic areas with poor sanitation.

What to do:

- Give an intramuscular dose of immune serum globulin (gamma globulin) of 0.02ml/kg.
- For prophylaxis of travelers who will be exposed longer than three months, use 0.05ml/kg, and instruct the patient to repeat this every 4 to 6 months.

What not to do:

- Do not withhold in pregnancy. Adverse reactions to human immune serum globulin are rare.

Discussion:

Immune serum globulin confers some immunity to hepatitis A (or at least modifies its course), but it is not adequate prophylaxis against hepatitis B and should be given in a larger dose (0.06ml/kg im) when used for post-needlestick prophylaxis of non-A non-B hepatitis.

Hepatitis B Prophylaxis

Presentation:

The patient has been exposed via blood from an infectious person (HBs Ag positive) on broken skin or mucous membranes, or has had sexual contact with an infectious person.

What to do:

- Ask whether the person exposed has been previously immunized against hepatitis B or, if the results are available within a

day, ascertain whether he already has adequate antibody levels (anti-HBs) and thus does not require immunization.
- If adequate anti-hepatitis B antibodies are not proven, provide passive immunity with hepatitis B immunoglobulin (HBIG) 0.06ml/kg im within 24–72 hours.
- Schedule a repeat dose of HBIG within 1 month, followed by an antibody (anti-HBs) level.

Discussion:

HBIG is quite expensive (and less necessary as hospital personnel are vaccinated against hepatitis B). The efficacy of passive immunity with HBIG falls off after 24–72 hours of exposure (sources differ, but HBIG is no longer effective after a week). Depending on laboratory services available, this may be time enough to verify whether the source is indeed HBsAg positive and the person exposed anti-HB negative (which is the only situation requiring passive immunity with HBIG).

Immune serum globulin (ISG), also known as gamma globulin, currently provides passive immunity almost as well as HBIG, and is much cheaper and more available. Identical doses of ISG may be substituted for HBIG above where HBIG is not available or affordable.

Needlestick

Presentation:

Someone in the hospital has been stuck by a needle, either from a patient with a known infection, from a patient of unknown infectiousness, or from no clear source, as when someone collecting the garbage feels himself stuck through the bag.

What to do:

- Clean the wound.
- Obtain HBsAg and VDRL results on the source, if possible, and baseline anti-HBs and VDRL on your patient.
- If your patient has not been successfully vaccinated against hepatitis B and the source is HBsAg positive or a high risk (e.g., a hepatitis or dialysis patient) give your patient hepatitis B immunoglobulin, 0.06ml/kg im, and make arrangements for a repeat dose in one month.

- If the source represents a low risk of hepatitis B (all other hospital needlesticks), give immune serum globulin 0.06ml/kg im.
- If the patient has not received a tetanus booster in the past five years, add Td or TT 0.5ml im.

Discussion:

Hepatitis B can be transmitted by infinitesimal quantities of blood, and requires expensive high titer passive immunity in the form of HBIG, largely because of the astronomical number of virus particles in infectious blood. It may be cost-effective to withhold HBIG in the emergency room, but if used it should be given early (best within one day, ineffective after seven) and it is hard to deny it to a co-worker in the hospital. The regimen above may overuse HBIG, but growing use of hepatitis B immunization will mitigate this common dilemma.

Acquired immunodeficiency syndrome (AIDS) is also becoming feared as a blood-borne infection hospital personnel can catch from patients: at present, the best we have to offer for prophylaxis is nonspecific immune serum globulin. ISG (gamma globulin) in the dose above is also the best we have for prophylaxis against cytomegalovirus and non-A non-B hepatitis, which are also commonly contracted from patient's blood. HBIG is simply ISG with a high titer of anti-HBs and thus provides the same general passive immunity as ISG (at greater cost).

Syphilis is also less contagious by needlestick—you have the option of giving prophylactic penicillin now, or waiting to see if the patient's VDRL turns positive.

Appendix

Digital Nerve Block

It is necessary to provide complete anesthesia when treating most fingertip injuries. Many techniques for performing a digital nerve block have been described. The following is one that is both effective and rapid in onset. This type of digital block will only provide anesthesia distal from the DIP joint but this is most often the site that demands a nerve block.

- Cleanse the finger and paint the area with povidone-iodine (Betadine) solution.
- Then, using a 27-gauge needle, inject 1% lidocaine midway between the dorsal and palmar surfaces of the finger at the midpoint of the middle phalanx.
- Initially, inject straight in along the side of the periosteum. Then pull back without removing the needle from the skin and fan the needle dorsally.
- Now advance the needle dorsally and inject again. Pull the needle back for the second time and without removing it from the skin, fan the needle in a palmar direction.
- Finally, advance the needle and inject the lidocaine in the vicinity of the digital neurovascular bundle. Always draw back to be sure your needle is not in the vessel. With each injection, instill enough xylocaine to produce visible soft tissue swelling—the actual number of cc's is not important.

To provide anesthesia on both sides of the fingertip, repeat this procedure on the opposite side of the finger. A similar block may be performed as far proximally as the middle of the metacarpal.

Do not use lidocaine (Xylocaine) with epinephrine. The digital arteries are end arteries that could potentially go into spasm and lead to an avascular necrosis of the fingertip (or at least to prolonged duration of anesthesia and to digital ischemia).

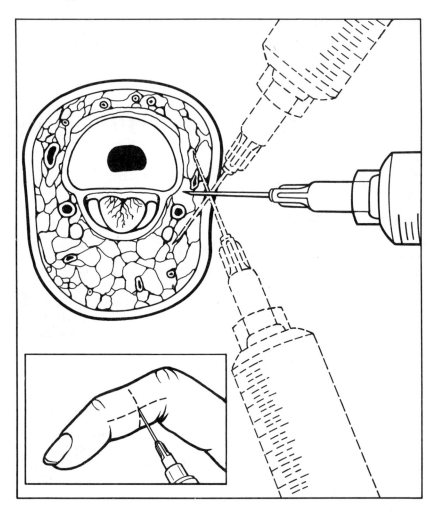

A Simple Finger Tip Dressing

To provide a complete non-adherent compression dressing for an injured fingertip, first cut out an L-shaped segment from a strip of oil emulsion (Adaptic) gauze. Cover the gauze with Betadine ointment to provide antiseptic protection as well as adhesion.

- Place the tip of the finger over the short leg of the gauze and then fold the gauze over the top of the finger.
- Now take the remaining leg and wrap it around the tip of the finger, resulting in a complete cover.

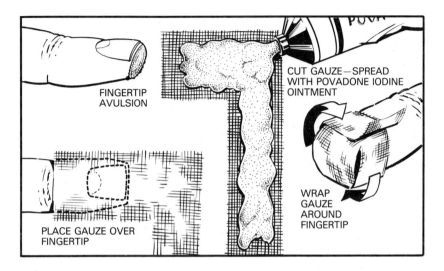

- For absorption and compression, fluff up a 4″ × 4″ cotton gauze pad and apply it over the entire end of the finger.
- Now cover this with either a Kling or tube gauze wrap and secure this with a spiral of adhesive tape.

    Do not place tight circumferential wraps of tape around a finger, especially if you anticipate swelling. This may act as a tourniquet and lead to vascular compromise. For this same reason use caution when applying tube gauze and do not use so much traction that the stockinette itself acts as a constricting band.

Complete Eye Exam

- visual acuity, using Snellen (wall) or Jaeger (hand-held) chart
- inspection of lids, conjunctivae, extraocular movement, pupillary reflexes
- visualization of retina, vessels, optic disc with ophthalmoscope
- slit lamp examination, with special attention to any blush of ciliary vessels at the corneal limbus (indicating iritis), any red cells (hyphema) or white cells (hypopyon) settling to the dependent arc of the anterior chamber, and any suspended white cells

or light flare (more signs of iritis) when the light is stopped down to a pinhole across the anterior chamber

- demonstration of the integrity of the corneal epithelium with fluorescein dye, which is taken up by corneal stroma or nonviable epithelium, and glows green under blue or ultraviolet light
- Note the depth of the anterior chamber using tangential lighting.

American Association of Poison Control Centers
Certified Regional Poison Centers

Arizona
Arizona Poison and Drug Information Center
Arizona Health Sciences Center
University of Arizona
Tucson, AZ 85724
602-626-6016 or 800-362-0101 (statewide)

California
University of California at Davis Medical Center
Regional Poison Center
2315 Stockton Boulevard
Sacramento, CA 95817
916-453-3692 or 800-852-7221 (Northern California)

San Diego Regional Poison Center
University of California Medical Center
225 West Dickinson Street
San Diego, CA 92103
619-294-6000

San Francisco Bay Area Regional Poison Center
San Francisco General Hospital
Room 1E 86
1001 Potrero Avenue
San Francisco, CA 94110
415-666-2845

Colorado
Rocky Mountain Poison Center
Denver General Hospital
West 8th & Cherokee Streets
Denver, CO 80204
303-629-1123 or 800-332-3073 (statewide)

District of Columbia
National Capital Poison Center
Georgetown University Hospital
3800 Reservoir Road, N.W.
Washington, DC 20007
202-625-3333

Florida
Tampa Bay Regional Poison Control Center
Tampa General Hospital
Davis Island
Tampa, FL 33606
813-251-6995 or 800-282-3171 (statewide)

Illinois
St. John's Hospital Regional Poison Resource Center
800 East Carpenter
Springfield, IL 62769
217-753-3330 or 800-252-2022 (statewide)

Indiana
Indiana Poison Center
1001 West Tenth Street
Indianapolis, IN 46202
317-630-7351 or 800-382-9097 (statewide)

Iowa   University of Iowa Hospitals and Clinics
                  Poison Control Center
                  Iowa City, IA 52242
                  319-356-2922 or 800-272-6477 (statewide)

Kentucky   Kentucky Regional Poison Center of Kosair-Children's
                     Hospital NKC, Inc.
                  P.O. Box 35070
                  Louisville, KY 40232
                  502-589-8222 or 800-722-5725 (statewide)

Maryland   Maryland Poison Center
                  20 North Pine Street
                  Baltimore, MD 21201
                  301-528-7701 or 800-492-2414 (statewide)

Michigan   Southeast Regional Poison Center
                  Children's Hospital of Michigan
                  3901 Beaubien
                  Detroit, MI 48201
                  313-494-5711 or 800-572-1655 (statewide)
                                 800-462-6642 (greater Detroit area)

Minnesota   Minnesota Poison Information Center
                  St. Paul-Ramsey Medical Center
                  640 Jackson Street
                  St. Paul, MN 55101
                  612-221-2113 or 800-222-1222 (statewide)

Nebraska   Mid-Plains Regional Poison Center
                  Children's Memorial Hospital
                  8301 Dodge
                  Omaha, NE 68114
                  402-390-5400 or 800-642-9999 (statewide)
                                 800-228-9515 (surrounding states)

New Jersey   New Jersey Poison Information and Education System
                  Beth Israel Medical Center
                  201 Lyons Avenue
                  Newark, NJ 07112
                  201-926-8005 or 800-962-1253 (statewide)

New Mexico   New Mexico Poison, Drug Information and Medical
                     Crisis Center
                  University of New Mexico
                  Albuquerque, NM 87131
                  505-843-2551 or 800-432-6866 (statewide)

New York   Long Island Regional Poison Center
                  Nassau County Medical Center
                  2201 Hempstead Turnpike
                  East Meadow, NY 11554
                  516-542-2324

New York City Regional Poison Center
Department of Health
Bureau of Laboratories
455 First Avenue
New York, NY 10016
212-340-4494 or 212-764-7667

Finger Lakes Poison Center
LIFELINE
University of Rochester Medical Center
Rochester, NY 14642
716-275-5151

Utah   Intermountain Regional Poison Control Center
50 North Medical Drive
Salt Lake City, UT 84132
801-581-2151

Drugs Referenced

GENERIC	BRAND	MANUFACTURER
acetic acid	Otic Domeboro Solution	Miles Pharmaceuticals
acetaminophen	Tylenol	McNeil Consumer Products
acyclovir	Zovirax	Burroughs Wellcome
aluminum hydroxide gel	Amphojel	Wyeth
antazoline & naphazoline	Vasocon-A	Smith, Miller & Patch
benzocaine etc	Cetacaine	Cetylite
benztropine	Cogentin	Merck Sharp & Dohme
betamethasone	Celestone, Valisone	Schering
bethanechol	Urecholine	Merck Sharp & Dohme
bismuth subsalicylate	Pepto-Bismol	Proctor & Gamble
bupivicaine	Marcaine	Breon
Burow's solution	Domeboro	Miles
carbamide peroxide	Debrox	Marion
cefadroxil	Duricef	Mead Johnson Pharmaceutical
cephalexin	Keflex	Dista
chlordiazepoxide	Librium	Roche
chlorpromazine	Thorazine	Smith Kline & French
clotrimazole	Lotrimin	Schering
codeine	Empirin with codeine	Burroughs Wellcome
	Tylenol with codeine	McNeil Pharmaceutical
colloidal oatmeal	Aveeno bath	CooperCare
crotamiton	Eurax	Westwood
cyclopentolate	Cyclogel	Alcon
cyproheptadine	Periactin	Merck Sharp & Dohme
dexamethasone	Decadron	Merck Sharp & Dohme
	Decaspray	Merck Sharp & Dohme
diazepam	Valium	Roche
diphenhydramine	Benadryl	Parke-Davis
diphenoxylate	Lomotil	Searle & Co.
ergotamine	Cafergot	Dorsey Pharmaceuticals

estrogens	Premarin	Ayerst
ethinyl estradiol	Norinyl	Syntex
& norethindrone	Ortho-Novum	Ortho Pharmaceutical
ethoxazene	Serenium	Squibb
fluocinonide	Lidex	Syntex
	Topsyn	Syntex
haloperidol	Haldol	McNeil Pharmaceutical
haloprogin	Halotex	Westwood
hydrocortisone	Anusol-HC/	Parke-Davis/Reed &
(primary ingredient)	Proctofoam-HC	Carnrick
suppositories & foam		
hydroxyzine	Atarax	Roerig
	Vistaril	Pfipharmecs
ibuprofen	Motrin	Upjohn
indomethacin	Indocin	Merck Sharp & Dohme
iodochlorhydroxyquin &	Vioform-	CIBA
hydrocortisone	Hydrocortisone	
kaolin & pectin	Kaopectate	Upjohn
lidocaine	Xylocaine	Astra
lindane	Kwell	Reed & Carnrick
loperamide	Imodium	Janssen
meclizine	Antivert	Roerig
medroxyprogesterone	Provera	Upjohn
mefenamic acid	Ponstel	Parke-Davis
meperidine	Demerol	Winthrop
methyldopa	Aldomet	Merck Sharp & Dohme
methylene blue etc	Trac Tabs	Hyrex
	Urised	Webcon
	Uroblue	Geneva
methylprednisolone	Medrol	Upjohn
metronidazole	Flagyl	Searle & Co.
miconazole	Monistat	Ortho
	Micatin	Ortho
microfibrillar collagen	Avitene	Alcon
naloxone	Narcan	Du Pont
naproxen	Anaprox	Syntex
	Naprosyn	Syntex
nystatin	Mycostatin	Squibb
	Nilstat	Lederle
oral protective paste	Orabase	Holloway
oxycodone	Percocet	Du Pont
	Percodan	Du Pont
phenazopyridine	Pyridium	Parke-Davis

GENERIC	BRAND	MANUFACTURER
phenol	Cepastat	Merrell Dow
	Chloraseptic	Proctor & Gamble
phenolphthalein	Ex-Lax	Ex-Lax
phenylbutazone	Butazolidin	Geigy
phenylephrine	Neo-Synephrine	Winthrop
phenytoin	Dilantin	Parke-Davis
povidone-iodine	Betadine	Purdue Frederick
prednisolone	Inflamase	Smith, Miller & Patch
prochlorperazine	Compazine	Smith Kline & French
pseudoephedrine	Sudafed	Burroughs Wellcome
psyllium	Metamucil	Searle Consumer Products
pyrantel pamoate	Antiminth	Pfipharmecs
pyrethrins, pyperonyl butoxide, etc	RID	Pfipharmecs
	R&C Spray III	Reed & Carnrick
	Li-Ban Spray	Pfipharmecs
scopolamine	Transderm-Scop	CIBA
selenium sulfide	Selsun	Abbott
silver sulfadiazene	Silvadene	Marion
sodium thiosulfate etc	Tinver	Barnes-Hind/ Hydrocurve
sulfamethoxazole & trimethoprim	Bactrim	Roche
	Septra	Burroughs Wellcome
sulfasoxazole	Gantrisin	Roche
tetanus immune globulin	Hypertet	Cutter
tetracaine	Pontocaine	Breon
tolnaftate	Aftate	Plough
	Tinactin	Schering
triamcinolone	Aristocort	Lederle
	Kenalog	Squibb
triethanolamine polypeptide oleate-condensate	Cerumenex	Purdue Frederick
witch hazel	Tucks	Parke-Davis

Index

Abductor pollicis longus tendon, 191
Abortion, spontaneous, 152–153
Abrasion, 233–235
Abscess, 256–257
  Bartholin's gland, 157–159
  cutaneous, 256–258
  dental, 98–99
  peritonsilar, 77
  rectal, 124
  retropharyngeal, 77
  subungual, 219
Absence, see Petit mal
Acetaminophen (Tylenol, Datril, Panadol, etc.), 104
Acetic acid (Otic Domeboro Solution), 56
Achilles tendon, 198–199
Acidosis, 8
Acoustic neuroma, 23,26
Acquired immunodeficiency syndrome, 282
Acrophobia, 22
Acyclovir (Zovirax), 91,142–143
Adrenaline, see Epinephrine
Aftate, see Tolnaftate
Agenda, 15
AIDS, see Acquired immunodeficiency syndrome
Akathisia, 12
Alcohol, see Ethanol
Aldomet, see Methyldopa
Alkalosis, 3,12
Allergy, 42–43,110,112–113,264–265
  anaphylaxis, 246–247,264
  angioedema, 264
  contact dermatitis, 239–240
  envenomation, 246–247
  neomycin, 32,57
  rhinitis, 73
  urticaria, 264–265
Alligator forceps, 56–57,61
Aluminum hydroxide gel (Amphojel), 124
Amblyomma americanum, 254–255
Ammonia, 2,8,10,113
Amnesia, 5
Amoxapine, 9
Amoxicillin, see Ampicillin

Amphetamine, 9
Amphojel, see Aluminum hydroxide gel
Ampicillin (and/or amoxicillin)
  for enterococcal UTI, 135,137
  for gonorrhea, 139,141
  rash with mononucleosis, 77,81
Amputation, fingertip, 203
Anaphylaxis, 246–247,264
Anaprox, see Naproxen
Anatomic snuffbox, 191
Anesthesia, local
  cornea, topical, 35,38,40,42,45–46,48
  digital block, 284–285
  for impalement, 230
  intercostal block, 108
  for procedures, 225,231,248,251,256,261
  spermatic cord, 144
  tetracaine-adrenaline-cocaine (TAC), 241
Angioedema, 264
Angle-closure glaucoma, 34
Antazoline & naphazoline (Vasocon-A), 31,43
Antihistamines, 74,104
Antiminth, see Pyrantel pamoate
Antivert, see Meclizine
Anusol-HC, see Hydrocortisone suppositories
Aphthous ulcer, 90
Aristocort, see Triamcinolone
Arterial blood gases, 3,106,112
Arthritis
  acute, 170–173
  degenerative, 171
  gonococcal, 140
  gout, 173
  bacterial, 171–172
  inflammatory, 172
  rheumatoid, 20
  temporomandibular joint, 83–85
  traumatic, 171
Aspirin (acetylsalicylic acid), 151,241,265
Asthma, 104
Atarax, see Hydroxyzine
Athlete's foot, 267–268
Aura, 7

Aveeno bath, *see* Colloidal
    oatmeal
Avulsion, extensor tendon, 196
Avulsion, finger tip, 203

Barb, removal, 230,231–233
Bartholin's gland abscess,
    157–159
Baseball finger, 196
Battle's sign, 5
Bacteria, *see* Infection
Bactrim, *see* Sulfamethoxazole &
    trimethoprim
BB shot, in skin, 251
Bee sting, 246–247
Bell's palsy, 27–28
Benadryl, *see* Diphenhydramine
Benzocaine (Cetacaine), 78
Benztropine (Cogentin), 12
Betadine, *see* Providone-iodine
Betamethasone (Celestone,
    Valisone), 174,239
Bethanechol (Urecholine), 147
Bicycle spoke injury, 222–223
Birth control pills, 152–153
Bismuth subsalicylate (Pepto-
    Bismol), 124
Bites, 235–237,278
Black eye, 29
"Black out," 1
Bleeding
    dental, 95
    hemorrhoids, 127
    nose, 66–68
    uterine, 153
    vaginal, 151–153
    rectal, 127–128
Blister, *see* Bulla or Vesicle
Blood poisoning, *see*
    Lymphangitis
Boil, 256–258
Bolt cutter, 210,230
Bone
    broken, *see* fracture
    caught in throat, 78
Borborygmi, 125
Bradycardia, 1
Brain tumor, 9,15,26,28

Bronchitis, 103,105
Bruises, 262–264
Bruxism, 83–85
Bugs, 59,253,271,273
Bullae, 242,245
Bupivicaine (Marcaine,
    Sensorcaine), 108
Burn
    sun, 240
    tar, 241–243
    thermal, 241–243
    tear gas, 110
    ultraviolet keratitis, 45–46
    welder's, 45–46
Burow's solution (Domeboro),
    239,241,270
Burr (ophthalmic instrument), 38
Bursitis, 172,174–175
Butazolidin, *see* Phenylbutazone
Butyrophenones, 12

Caffeine, 15
Caffergot, *see* Ergotamine
Cast spreader, 210
Candidiasis
    diaper rash, 275
    oral, 101
    vaginitis, 154–156
Canker sore, 90
Carbamide peroxide (Debrox), 54
Carbon dioxide, 5% (Carbogen), 3
Carbon monoxide, 15,25,112–113
Carpal navicular, 191
Carpal tunnel syndrome, 188–190
Carpopedal spasm, 2,4
Cautery, 66–67,214–215,260
Cefoxatin, 142
Celestone, *see* Betamethasone
Cellulitis, 43,258–260
Cepastat, *see* Phenol
Cephalgia (headache), 14–19
Cerebrospinal fluid, 5,75
Cerumen impaction, 53–54
Cerumenex, *see* Triethanolamine
    polypeptide oleate-
    condensate
Cervical strain, 161–162
Cervicitis, 140,154

Cetacaine, see Benzocaine
Chalazion, 47
Cheiralgia paresthetica, 186–188
Chemosis, 42
Chickenpox, precursor of
  shingles, 270
Chin, caught in zipper, 260
Chip fracture, 194
Chlamydia, 139–141,144
Chloraseptic, see Phenol
Chlorpromazine (Thorazine),
  19,115
Chorionic gonadotropin, see
  Human chorionic
  gonadotropin
Circumcision, 148,262
"Clap," 140–142
Clotrimazole (Lotrimin,
  Mycelex), 101,154,268,276
"Clue cells" of Gardnerella
  vaginitis, 154
CMV, see Cytomegalovirus
Cocaine, 9,66,71,72,241
Coccyx fracture, 166–168
Codeine, 104, 265
Cogentin, see Benztropine
Colchicine, 172,173
Cold, 103–105
Cold sore, 90–91
Colloidal oatmeal (Aveeno bath) 239
Colorful urine, 138–139
Coma
  hysterical, 9
  removal of hard contact lenses
    in, 50–51
Compazine, see Prochlorperazine
Computed tomography (CT),
  6,9,15,17
Concussion, 5
Conjunctivitis, 5
Constipation, 125–126
Contact dermatitis, 239–240
Contact lenses, 42,47–51
Contraceptive pills, 152–153
Contusions, 262–264
Conversion reaction, 9
Convulsion, 7
"Cooties," 271
Cornea, 35–41,45–46,47–48
  abrasion, 40–41
  foreign body in, 38–39

Costochondral separation, 105
Costochondritis, 108–109
Coudé catheter, 146
Cough, 103–104,110–113,119
Crab lice, 271
Cramp
  menstrual, 151–152
  muscle, 151,165,168–170
Crotamiton (Eurax), 274
CSF, see Cerebrospinal fluid
CT, see Computed tomography
Cubital tunnel syndrome, 190
Cultures
  conjunctival, 32
  for gonorrhea, 141
  for herpes, 142
  stool, 124–125
  urethral, 139–141
  urine, 136–137
Cutaneous abscess or pustule,
  256–258
Cyclogel, see Cyclopentolate
Cyclopentolate (Cyclogel), 34
Cyproheptadine (Periactin), 264
Cyst, ganglion, 190
Cystitis, 135–136
Cytomegalovirus, 81

Debridment, 203–204,234–235,
  242–244
Debrox, see Carbamide peroxide
Decadron, see Dexamethasone
Decaspray, see Dexamethasone
Demerol, see Meperidine
Dental pain, 96–100
Dental surgery, complications,
  95–97
Dental trauma, 94–95
DeQuervain's tenosynovitis, 187
Dermabrasion, 234–235,250,254
Dermacentor andersoni &
  variabilis, 254–255
Dexamethasone (Decadron,
  Decaspray, Hexadrol), 241
Dextromethorphan, 104
Diaper rash, 275–276
Diarrhea, 123–125
Diazepam (Valium), 7,12

Dilantin, *see* Phenytoin
Diphenhydramine (Benadryl), 12
Diphenoxylate (Lomotil), 122,124
Diptheria, 77
Disc, intervertebral, 163,165–166
Discharge
  nasal, 69,73,103
  phimosis, 148
  rectal, 140
  urethral, 139–142
  vaginal, 154–156
Dislocation
  contact lens, 49–50
  elbow, 180–181
  finger, 194–195
  jaw, 86–87
  nail, 205–206
  spine, 163,165–166
Disulfiram-like action of
    metronidazole, 154
Dizziness, 22,83
DJD, *see* Arthritis, degenerative
Domeboro, *see* Burow's solution
Domeboro Otic, *see* Acetic acid
"Drip," 139–142
Drooling, 27,116
Drug-seeking patients, 18
Dry socket, 96–97
DUB, *see* Dysfunctional uterine
    bleeding
Dysentery, 123–125
Dysfunctional uterine bleeding,
    153
Dyskinesias, 12
Dysmenorrhea, 151–152
Dysphagia, 75
Dyspnea, 2,108
Dystonias, 12
Dysuria, 135,137,139,140,147,154

Ear, 53–65
  blocked, 53–54
  congested, 61–63
  drum, 58,62–64
  foreign body in, 59–60
  frostbite, 245
  glue, 64
  infection, canal, 55–57

irrigation, 53–62
lacerated, 65
lobe, 65,245
pain, 55,58,61
ringing in, *see* Tinnitus
swimmer's, 55–57
swollen, 42–43
wax, 53–54
Earring, 65
Ectopic pregnancy, 153,166
Edema
  arthritis, 170
  burn, 240
  bursitis, 174
  calf swelling, 198
  conjunctival, 42
  contusion, 262
  envenomation, 246
  finger, 209
  ligament, 176
  muscle, 177
  joint effusion, 178
  periorbital, 42
  rewarming, 245
  urticaria, 264
Effusion, 171–172,178–179
Elbow, 180–183
Enterobiasis, 126–127
Envenomation, 246–247
Epididymitis, 143–144
Epiglottitis, 77
Epilepsy, 8–11
Epinephrine, 241,283,264
Epistaxis, 66–68
Eponychium, 205–208,213,
    219–221
Ergotamine (Cafergot, Gynergen,
    etc.), 17
Erysipelas, 258–260
Erythrocyte sedimentation rate,
    19,169
Esophageal food bolus
    obstruction, 116
ESR, *see* Erythrocyte
    sedimentation rate
Estrogens (Premarin, etc.), 153
Ethanol (ethyl alcohol), 8,265
Ethinyl estradiol &
    norethindrone (Norinyl,
    Ortho-Novum, etc.), 153
Ethoxazene (Serenium), 138

Eugenol, 97,99
Eurax, see Crotamiton
Eustachian tube, 63–64
Ewald tube, 116
Ex-Lax, see Phenolphthalein
Extensor pollicis longus & brevis
    tendons, 191
Extensor tendon avulsion—distal
    phalanx, 196–198
Eye, 29–51
    black, 29–30
    contact lenses, 47–51
    foreign body in, 35–39
    infection, 31–32,46–47
    injury, 29–30,35–41
    lid, 35–37,46–47,50–51
    pain, 32–41,45–46,47–48
    red, 31–35,44–46
Eyestrain, headache, 15

Facette, 163–166
Faint, 1
"Fall out," 1
Fat pad sign on x ray, 183,191
FB, see Foreign body
Fecal leukocytes, 124
Felon, 221
Fever, 15,55,74,76,80,104,124,135,
    137,144,145,253–256,258
Fibromyalgia, 168–170
Finger, 194–198
Fingernail, see Nail
Fingernail avulsion, 207–209
Fingertip amputation, 203
Fishhook removal, 231–233
"Fishy" odor of Gardnerella
    vaginitis, 154
"Fits," 7
Flagyl, see Metronidazole
Flank pain, 137
Fluocinonide (Lidex, Topsyn), 239
Fluorescein dye, 29,31,34,35,36,
    39,40,42,44,45,48,49,110
Fluttering eyelids, 10
Foley catheter, 68,70,119,130,146
Foot, 222–229,245,267–268
Foreign body
    BB shot, 251

cerumen impaction, 53–54
circumferential, 209
conjunctival, 35–37
contact lens, 49–50
corneal, 38–39
ear, 59–60
esophageal, 116–120
eye, 35–39
fingernail, 217–218
fishhook, 231–232
foot (needle), 223–226
metallic, 251–252
needle, 223–226
nose, 69–71
rectal, 129–133
ring, 209–211,247
in skin, 246–256
sliver, superficial, 247–248
subungual, 217–218
swallowed, 119–120
throat, 78–79
tick head, 254
vaginal, 156–157
x rays for locating,
    223–231,250–253
Foreskin, 148–149,260–262
Fracture
    blowout, 29
    carpal navicular, 191–193
    coccyx, 166–168
    elbow, 182
    finger, 194–197,203–208
    neck, 161
    nose, 72
    radius, 182–184
    rib, 105–108
    scaphoid, 191–193
    skull, 5, 29
    tail, 166
    toe, 200–201
    tooth, 94
    wrist, 191
    zygoma, 29
Frenulum, 88
Frequency, urinary, 135,137,
    144,145
Frostbite, 244–245
Frostnip, 244–245
Fungus, 56,267–268

Gamekeeper's thumb, 193
Gamma globulin, see Globulin
Ganglion cyst, 190–191
Gantrisin, see Sulfasoxazole
Gastrocnemius tear, 199
Gardnerella, 154–156
Germinal matrix, 208,213
Giemsa stain, 91,142
Gingivitis, 100
Gland
    Bartholin's, 158
    lymph, see Lymphadenopathy
    meibomian (eyelid), 47
    Moll (eyelid), 47
    parotid, 92–93
    prostate, 145
    salivary, 91–93
    sebaceous, 54
    sublingual, 93
    submaxillary, 92–93
    sweat, eccrine & apocrine, 258
    Zeiss (eyelid), 47
Glandular fever, 80
Glaucoma, acute angle-closure,
    34
Globulin, immune serum (ISG),
    280–282
    hepatitis B immune globulin
        (HBIG) (Hyperhep, etc),
        280–281
    rabies immune globulin (RIG)
        (Hyperab, etc.), 278–279
    tetanus immune globulin (TIG)
        (Hypertet, etc.), 277–278
Globus hystericus, 80
Glomerulonephritis, post-
    streptococcal, 77
Glucagon, 116
Gonadotropin, see Human
    chorionic gonadotropin
Gonorrhea, 144,154,158
    pharyngeal, 76
    urethral, 139–142
"Goose egg," 5
Gout, 173
Gram stain, 101,124,135,137,
    139–141,171,174
Grand mal, 7
Granulation tissue, 259–260
Guillain-Barré syndrome, 21

Haldol, see Haloperidol
Haloperidol (Haldol), 12
Haloprogin (Halotex), 268
Halotex, see Haloprogin
Hand, 184–198,203–221,230–237,
    247,258,273,283–285
Hand-foot-and-mouth disease, 90
Handcuff neuropathy, 186–187
HBIG, see Globulin, hepatitis B
    immune
hCG, see Human chorionic
    gonadotropin
HDCV, see Human diploid cell
    vaccine
Headache
    caffeine withdrawal, 16
    cluster, 18
    eyestrain (refraction), 15
    dysmenorrhea, 151
    migraine, 15
    muscle tension, 14
    sinusitis, 73
    temperomandibular joint, 83
    temporal arteritis, 19
Head trauma, 5
Hearing, 53–54,62–64
Heart attack, 108–110,116
Hematoma
    contusions, 262–264
    muscle tear, 177
    periorbital, 29
    septal, 72
    scalp, 5,6
    subconjunctival, 29,44–45
    subdural, 6
    subungual, 214–215
Hematuria, 135,147
Hemorrhagic cystitis, 135
Hemorrhoids, 127–129
Hemotympanum, 5
Hepatitis
    hepatitis A, 280
    hepatitis B, 280–282
    hepatitis, non-A, non-B, 282
    hepatitis B immune globulin
        (HBIG), 280–282
Herald patch, 265–267
Herpangina, 90
Herpes
    keratitis, 32,35

simplex, genital, 142–143,147
simplex, oral, 90–91
varicella-zoster (shingles), 28,269–270
zoster ophthalmicus, 270
Hiccups, 115–116
Hives, 264–265
Hordeolum, 46–47
Human chorionic gonadotropin, 151–152,154
Human diploid cell vaccine (for rabies), 279
Hydrocortisone
   in suppositories (Anusol-HC, etc.), 128
   in rectal foam (Proctofoam-HC, etc.), 128
   and iodochlorhydroxyquin (Vioform-Hydrocortisone), 268
Hydroxyzine (Vistaril, Atarax), 43,239,264
Hymenoptera envenomation, 246
Hyperab, see Globulin, immune serum
Hyperhep, see Globulin, immune serum
Hypertet, see Globulin, immune serum
Hyperventilation, 2
Hyphema, 29
Hysteria, 9–11

Ibuprofin (Motrin, Nuprin, Rufen, etc.), 22,42,108,162,165
Ice, 165,176,178,183,191,193,196, 198,200,243,246,263
Imodium, see Loperamide
Impalement, 229–231
Impetigo, 274–275
Indomethacin (Indocin), 151,173
Infection
   candida, 101,155,275
   conjunctivitis, 31–32
   dental, 97–98
   dermatophyte, 267–268
   diarrhea, 123–125
   hand, 258

hepatitis, 280–281
herpes, 90–91,142–143,269–270
joint, 171,172
mononucleosis, 80–81
oral, 100–101
pharyngitis, 75–77
sinusitis, 73–75
skin, 256–260
staphlococcal, 123,259,275
streptococcal, 76–77,259
upper respiratory, 103–105
Infestation, 126,271–274
Inflamase, see Prednisolone
Inflammation
   bursa, 174
   joint, 170
   muscle, 19
   skin, 239–47, 264–275
Ingrown toenail, 219
Insect bite, 246
Insects on skin, 253,271,273
Iodochlorhydroxyquin & hydrocortisone (Vioform-Hydrocortisone), 268
Ipecac, syrup of, 119–121
Iritis, 32–35
ISG, see Globulin, immune serum
Itch, see Pruritis
Ixodes dammini, 254–255

Jaw, 83–87
Jock itch, 267–268
Joint
   dislocation, see Dislocation
   effusion, 178–179
   fluid, 171
   infection, 171–172
   injury, 176–177
   subluxation, 180
   temporomandibular, 83–87

Kaolin & pectin (Kaopectate, Peripectolin, etc.), 124
Kaopectate, see Kaolin & pectin
Kenalog, see Triamcinolone

Keratoconjunctivitis, 32,45–46
Kiesselbach's area, 66
KOH, see Potassium hydroxide
Kwell, see Lindane

Labrynthitis, 25,26
Lead poisoning from pencil
    point, 250
Leukocytes
    in joint fluid, 171–172
    in diarrhea stool, 124
    in infected urine, 135–137
    in tubular casts, 137
Li-Ban Spray, see Pyrethrins,
    piperonyl butoxide, etc.
Lice, 271
Lidex, see Fluocinonide
Lidocaine (Xylocaine, etc.), 9,76,
    78,109,170
Ligament sprains, 176–177,
    193–195
Lightheaded, 1,22
Limbal blush, 32–33
Lindane (Kwell, Scabene), 272
LOC, see loss of consciousness
Lomotil, see Diphenoxylate
Loperamide (Imodium), 122,124
Loss of consciousness, 2,5
Lotrimin, see Clotrimazole
Louse, 271
Ludwig's angina, 99
Lumbar strain, 165
Lyme disease, 254
Lymphadenopathy, 75,80,103,258
Lymphangitis, 246,256,258–259

Mace, 110–111
Major impalement injuries, 231
Mallet finger, 196
Mandible, 83–87
Marcaine, see Bupivicaine
Mast cells, 265
Meat impaction, 116
Meclizine (Antivert, Bonine, etc.),
    23

Median nerve compression,
    188–190
Medrol, see Methylprednisolone
Mefanamic acid (Ponstel), 151
Meibomian gland, 47
Meibomianitis, 46–47
Ménière's disease, 23,26
Meningitis, 6,15
Menorrhagia, 152
Menses, 151–153
Menstrual cramps, 151–152
Meperidine (Demerol, Mepergan),
    18,242
Metallic foreign body, 251–253
Metamucil, see Psyllium
Methyldopa (Aldomet, etc.), 138
Methylene blue (in Trac Tabs,
    Urised, Uroblue, etc.), 138
Methylprednisolone (Medrol,
    etc.), 109,170
Metronidazole (Flagyl, etc.), 139,
    154–155
Metrorrhagia, 152
Micatin, see Miconazole
Miconazole (Monistat, Micatin),
    154,268
Migraine headache, 17
Minor impalement injuries,
    229–231
Miscarriage, 152–153
Mites, 273–274
Monistat, see Miconazole
Mononucleosis, 76,80–81
Motrin, see Ibuprofen
Mouth
    infections, 90–91,100–101
    laceration, 87–90
    salivary stones, 91–93
    sores, 90–91
Mucin clot, 171
Multinucleate giant cell, 91,142
Mumps, 93
Muscle
    cricopharyngeus, 80,120
    gastrocnemius, 199
    gluteus medius, 169
    infraspinatus, 169
    levator scapulae, 163
    occipitalis, 15,163
    plantaris, 198–199

quadratus lumborum, 169–170
rectus abdominus, 122
semispinalis, 169
splenius, 163,169
sternocleidomastoid, 163,169
temporalis, 15
trapezius, 163,169
Muscle strains, 177–178
Myalgia, 15,19,80,103,164,168
Mycoplasma pneumonia, 104
Mycostatin, see Nystatin
Myofascial pain syndrome, 14,168
Myocardial infarction, 108–110,
    116

Nail, finger or toe, 205–209,
    212–221
Nail avulsion, 207–209
Nail infection, 219–221
Nail root dislocation, 205–209
Nail, stepped on, 227,229
Nail trephination, hot paper clip
    for, 220–221
Nailbed laceration, 212–213
Naprosyn, see Naproxen
Naproxen (Anaprox, Naprosyn),
    151,170
Nausea, 5,17,121–123,137,
    144,151,240
Neck, 161–165
Needle in foot, 223–226
Neomycin, reaction to, 32,57
Neo-Synephrine, see
    Phenylephrine
Nerve
  cervical roots, 161,163
  digital, 283–284
  dorsal ganglia, 270
  facial, 28
  glossopharyngeal, 116
  lumbar roots, 165
  median, 188–189
  phrenic, 115
  radial, 184–187
  trigeminal, 28
Nilstat, see Nystatin
Nits, 271–272

Norinyl, see Ethinyl estradiol &
    norethindrone
Nose, 66–74
  bleed, 66–68
  broken, 72–73
  discharge, 69,73,103
  foreign body in, 69–71
  frostbite, 245
  irrigation of, 70–71,73–74
Numbness, see Paresthesia
Nursemaid's elbow, 180–182
Nystagmus, 22
Nystatin (Micostatin, Nilstat),
    101,164,275

Oculogyric crisis, 12
Odynophagia, 75
Oil of cloves, 97,99
Opisthotones, 12
Orabase, see Oral protective paste
Oral protective paste (Orabase),
    90,91
Ortho-Novum, see Ethinyl
    estradiol & norethindrone
Orthostatic hypotension, 2
Osteoarthritis, 171
Otic Domeboro solution, see
    Acetic acid
Otitis
  externa, 55–57,83
  serous, 61,103
Oxycodone (Percocet, Percodan,
    Tylox, etc.), 42,45,47,242,270

PABA, see Para-aminobenzoic
    acid, 241
Pain
  abdominal, 121–126,140,144,
    146,151,170,269
  back, 137,145,151,165–168,151
  burn, 241–242
  chest, 105–110,269
  ear, 55,58,61
  eye, 32–41,45–46,47–48
  dental, 96–99
  face, 83,269

flank, 137,144,170,269
gas, 125–126
headache, 14–18
herpes, 90,269
muscle, 15,19,80,103,164,168
neck, 161–164,269
perineal, 145,157
rectal, 127–128,140,166
scrotal, 144
subungual hematoma, 214–215
suprapubic, 135,146,151
thigh, 151,165
trigger points, 168–170
Paint chip under nail, 217
Paper clip as x ray skin marker,
    223–225
Para-aminobenzoic acid, 241
Paralysis
    facial, 27–28
    hysterical, 9–11
    radial neuropraxia, 184–185
Paraphimosis, 148–149
Paresthesia, 2,27,269
Parkinsonism, 12
Paronychia, 219–221
Partial thickness burn, 241–244
Pectin & kaolin (Kaopectate,
    Peripectolin, etc.), 124
Pediculosis, 271–272
Pediculus capitis, 271
Pencil point puncture, 249–250
Penicillin, 76,99,139,141,275
Penis, 139–142,146–149,260–262
Pepto-Bismol, see Bismuth
    subsalicylate
Percocet, see Oxycodone
Percodan, see Oxycodone
Periactin, see Cyproheptadine
Period, menstrual, 151–153
Petit mal, 7
pH, in diagnosis of vaginitis, 154
Phalen's test, 188–189
Pharyngitis, 75–77,142
Phenazopyridine (Pyridiom, etc.),
    135,138–139
Phencyclidine, 9
Phenol (Cepastat, Chloraseptic,
    etc.), 76
Phenolphthalein (Ex-Lax, etc.),
    138

Phenothiazines, 12,241
Phenylbutazone (Butazolidin)
Phenylephrine (Neo-Synephrine,
    etc.), 63,66,69,72,74,104
Phenytoin (Dilantin), 8
Phimosis, 148–149
Pin cutter, 210,230
Pinworms, 126–127
PIP joint, see Proximal
    interphalangeal joint
Piperonyl butoxide, see
    Pyrethrins, piperonyl
    butoxide, etc.
Pityriasis rosea, 265–267
Plantaris tendon rupture, 198–199
PMR, see Polymyalgia
    rheumatica
Pneumonia, 3
Pneumothorax. 3,78,105,108
Podagra, 173
Poison
    control centers, 120–121,
        287–289
    food, 121–123
    gas, 111–113
    ivy, oak, & sumac, 239–240
Polymyositis, 20
Polymyalgia rheumatica, 19
Ponstel, see Mefenamic acid
Pontocaine, see Tetracaine
Pope ear wick, 56
Postictal period, 7
Potassium hydroxide prep, 154,
    268
Povidone-iodine (Betadine, etc.),
    155
Prednisolone (Inflamase), 34
Prednisone, 19,27,239,241,270
Pregnancy test, 151–152,154
Premarin, see Estrogens
Probenecid, 136,139,141
Prochlorperazine (Compazine),
    122
Proctofoam-HC, see
    Hydrocortisone foam
Prostaglandins, 151
Prostatitis, 145
Proud flesh, 259–260
Proximal intephalangeal joint
    dislocation, 194–196

Pruritis, 83,126,239–240,264–274
Pseudoephedrine (Sudafed, etc.),
    63,74,104
Pseudoseizures, 8–11
Psyllium (Metamucil, etc.),
    124–126,129
Pthirus pubis, 271
Ptomaine, 121
Pulmonary embolus, 3
Pulpitis, 97
Puncture wound, 223–233,236,
    247–253,277–278,281–282
Pus, 73,157,220,249,252,256–258
Pustule, 256–258
Pyelonephritis, 137,166
Pyogenic granuloma, 259–260
Pyrantel pamoate (Antiminth),
    127
Pyrethrins, piperonyl butoxide,
    etc. (R&C Spray III, Li-Ban
    Spray), 272
Pyridium, see Phenazopyridine

R&C Spray III, see Pyrethrins,
    piperonyl butoxide, etc.
Rabies, prophylaxis, 77,278–279
Raccoon eyes, 5
Radial head fracture, 182–184
Radial neuropathy, 184–186
Range of motion, 161,162–164,
    174,176,178,180
Rash, 76,80,140,239–240,264–276
Rectal exam, 124–133,145–147,
    166–167
Reduction, see Dislocation
Rewarming, 245
Rheumatic fever, 77
Rhinitis, 103
    allergic, 73
    medicamentosa, 64,74
Rhus dermatitis, 239–240
Rib
    belt, 105–108
    broken, 105–108
    inflamed, 108–110
RID, see Pyrethrins, piperonyl
    butoxide, etc.
RIG, see Globulin, rabies immune
Ring removal, 209–211

Ringer's lactate, 122
Ringworm, 267–268
Rinne test, 63
RMSF, see Rocky mountain
    spotted fever
"Road rash," 233–235
Rocky mountain spotted fever,
    254
ROM, see Range of motion
Rust ring (from metallic corneal
    foreign body), 38

Salicylates, 3
Saliva, 78,116,278
Salivary duct stones, 91–93
Sarcoptes scabiei, 274
Saturday night palsy, 184
Saucerization to debride
    puncture wound, 227–229
Scabies, 273,274
Scaphoid fracture, 191–193
Schatzki's ring, 118
Scopolamine (Transderm-Scop),
    25
Scotoma, 17
Second-degree burn, 241–244
Seizures, 7
    alcohol withdrawal, 8
    epilepsy, 8
    hysterical, 9
    overdose, 9
    psychomotor, 11
    traumatic, 5
Septra, see Sulfamethoxazole &
    trimethoprim
Serenium, see Ethoxazene
Serous otitis media, 62–64
Shingles, 269–270
Shortness of breath, see Dyspnea
Sialolithiasis, 91–93
Sighing, 2
Silvadene, see Silver sulfadiazene
Silver sulfadiazene (Silvadene),
    242
Singultus, 73–75
Sinusitis, 115–116
Skin graft, 203–205
Skipole thumb, 193
Slit lamp exam, 33,35,38

Sliver under nail, 217–218
Sliver under skin, 247–249
Smelling salts, 8
Smoke inhalation, 111–113
SOB, *see* Shortness of breath
Sodium thiosulfate, etc. (Tinver), 268
Soft collar, 162,164
Sore throat, 75–77
"Spaghetti & meatballs" appearance on KOH prep, 154,268
Spasm, 2,5,14,162–166
Spectinomycin, 139,141
Spica, 192–193
Splint, 174,176–178,183,185,187, 188,191–197,200–201,263
Splinter, *see* Sliver
Spoke injury, 222–223
Sprain, 161–162,165–166, 176–177,192
Spud (ophthalmic instrument), 38
Staphlococcal food poisoning, 121
Status epilepticus, 7
Steakhouse syndrome, 116
Stenson's duct, 92
Stiff neck, 6,15,161–165
Sting, 246
Strain, 161–162,165–166,177–178
Streptococcal pharyngitis, 76
String test, 171
Strychnine, 12
Sty, 46–47
Subconjunctival hemorrhage, 29
Subluxation of the head of the radius, 180–182
Subungual ecchymosis, 216
Subungual foreign body, 217–218
Subungual hematoma, 214–216
Sudafed, *see* Pseudoephedrine
Sulfadiazene, silver, *see* Silver sulfadiazene
Sulfamethoxazole & trimethoprim (Bactrim, Septra), 135,137,145
Sulfasoxazole (Gantrisin, etc.), 135,137
Sulfonamide photosensitivity, 241
Sunscreens, 241

Superficial finger tip avulsion, 203–205
Superficial sliver, 247–248
Supraglottitis, 77
Swallowed foreign body, 119–120
Swelling, *see* Edema
Swimmer's ear, 55–57
Swoon, 1
Syncope, 1
Syndrome
  Guillain-Barré, 21
  hyperventilation, 2
  Kawasaki's, 31
  Reiter's, 31
  Stevens-Johnson, 31
Synovial fluid, 171–172
Syphilis, 139–142,266–267

TAC, *see* Tetracaine-adrenaline-cocaine, 234
Tailbone fracture, 166–168
Tar burn, 241–242
Tar removal, 244
Tarsal plate, eyelid, 36–37,46–47
Tattoos, traumatic, 233–235
TD, Td, 278
Tear gas, 110–111
Teeth, 94–100
  broken, 94–95
  knocked out, 94–95
  loosened, 94–95
  painful, 97–100
Temporal arteritis, 20
Temporomandibular joint arthritis, 83–86
Tendon injuries, 177–178,196–199
Tendon sheath, 190–191
Tenesmus, 123,140
Tension headache, 14
Tennis elbow, 184
Tennis leg, 199
Testicle, torsion, 144
Tetanus, prophylaxis, 12,277–278
Tetanus toxoid, 278
Tetracaine (Pontocaine, Cetacaine), 46,66,69,72,241
Tetracaine-adrenaline-cocaine topical anesthesia, 241

Tetracycline, 139–141,144–145,241
Thayer-Martin culture medium,
    140–142,154
Thiazide photosensitivity, 241
Thiosulfate, sodium, see Sodium
    thiosulfate
Thorazine, see Chlorpromazine
Threadworms, 126–127
Throat, 75–81
  foreign body in, 78–80
  sore, 75–77,80–81
  strep, 76
Thrush, 101
Thumb, 184–194
Tick, 253–256
TIG, see Globulin, tetanus
    immune
Tinactin, see Tolnaftate
Tinea, 267–269
Tinel's sign, 188
Tingling, see Paresthesia
Tinnitus, 53,58,62,83
Tinver, see Sodium thiosulfate
    etc.
TM, see Tympanic membrane or
    Ear drum
TMJ, see Temporomandibular
    joint
Toe, 173,200–201,205–208,219–221
Toenail, see Nail
Toenail avulsion, 207–209
Tolnaftate (Aftate, Tinactin, etc.),
    268
Tonsillitis, 77
Topsyn, see Fluocinonide
Torsion, testicular, 144
Torticollis, 12,162–164
Tourniquet, 209,213,225
Toxic screen, 8
Toxicodendron, see Rhus
Trac Tabs, see Methylene blue
Transderm-Scop, see
    Scopolamine
Traumatic effusion, 178–179
Trephination of nail, 214
Triamcinolone (Aristocort,
    Kenalog), 239
Trichomonas, 136,139,154–156
Triethanolamine polypeptide
    oleate-condensate
    (Cerumenex), 54

"Trigger points," 168
Trimethoprim, see
    Sulfamethoxazole &
    trimethoprim
Trismus, 83,86,99
TT, 278
Tucks, see Witch hazel
Tylenol, see Acetaminophen
Tympanic membrane, 58,62–64,
    115
Tzanck prep, 91,142

Ulnar collateral ligament tear,
    193–194
Ultraviolet keratoconjunctivitis,
    45–46
Unconscious
  from head trauma, 2,161
  removal of contact lenses
      when, 50–51
Upper respiratory infection,
    103–105
Urecholine, see Bethanechol
Urgency, urinary, 135,137,145,
    146,154
URI, see Upper respiratory
    infection
Uric acid, 171–173
Urinary obstruction, 145–147
Urinary retention, 146–147
Urinary tract infection,
    135–137,139–145
  lower tract, 135–136
  upper tract, 137
Urine, colorful, 138–139
Urised, see Methylene blue
Uroblue, see Methylene blue
Urticaria, 264–265
UTI, see Urinary tract infection
Uveitis, anterior, 32

Vaginal bleeding, 152–153
Vaginal foreign body, 156–157
Vaginitis, 135,154–156
Valisone, see Betamethasone
Valium, see Diazepam

Vasocon-A, *see* Antazoline & naphazoline
Vasovagal syncope, 1–2
VDRL, 139–142,266–267,281–282
Venom, 247
Vermillion border, 89
Vernal conjunctivitis, 31
Vertigo, 17,22
Vesicles, 90,142,239–245
Vestibular neuronitis, 25,26
Vinegar, 155
Vioform-hydrocortisone, *see* Iodochlorhydroxyquin & hydrocortisone
Virus, *see* Infection
Vistaril, *see* Hydroxizine
Vitamin C for colds, 105
Volar plate, 196
Vomiting, 6,15,119–123,137,151

Wasp sting, 246–247
WaterPik®, 54,59–60
Weakness, 17,19–22
    face, 27
Welts, 264
Wharton's duct, 92
Wheals, 264
Whiplash, 161–162
White blood cells, *see* Leukocytes
Witch hazel (Tucks), 129
Wisdom tooth, 99
Word catheter, 157–159
"Worst headache," 15
Wright's stain, 91,124,142
Wrist, 184–194
Wrist drop, 184
Wry neck, 162–163

X rays
    abdominal, 130,133
    acute arthritis, 171
    barium swallow, 79,116,119
    bicycle spoke injury of foot, 223
    chest, 108,109,112,115
    for contusions, pain, swelling, 263
    coccyx, 167
    crosstable lateral cervical spine, 161
    CT, *see* Computed tomography
    dental, 93
    extensor tendon avulsion, 197
    finger dislocations, 194
    fingertip crush, 203
    ganglion cyst, 190
    for gas in cellulitis, 259
    with impaled objects, 230
    IVP, 137
    ligament sprains, 176
    lumbosacral, 164–166
    nail injuries, 205–207
    neck, 161–162
    nose, 72
    nursemaid's elbow, 182
    plantaris tendon rupture, 199
    radial head fracture, 183–184
    rib fractures, 105
    salivary stones, 93
    scaphoid fracture, 191–193
    sinuses, 73
    skull, 5,8,30
    soft tissue for FB, 79,119,250
    toe fracture, 200
    traumatic effusions, 178
    ulnar collateral ligament of thumb, 193
    xerogram, 250
Xylocaine, *see* Lidocaine
Xyphoid cartilage, 109

Yeast, 101,155,275

Zenker's diverticulum, 79
Zipper, 260–262
Zovirax, *see* Acyclovir